THE
100
MOST BEAUTIFUL
BIRDS
IN THE WORLD

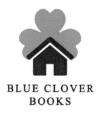

**BLUE CLOVER
BOOKS**

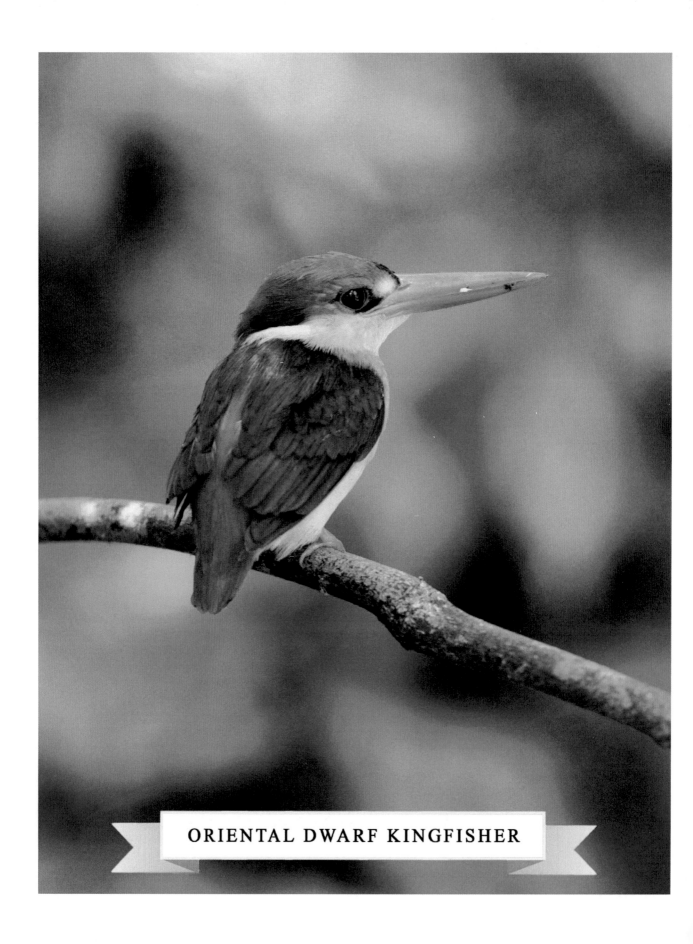

ORIENTAL DWARF KINGFISHER

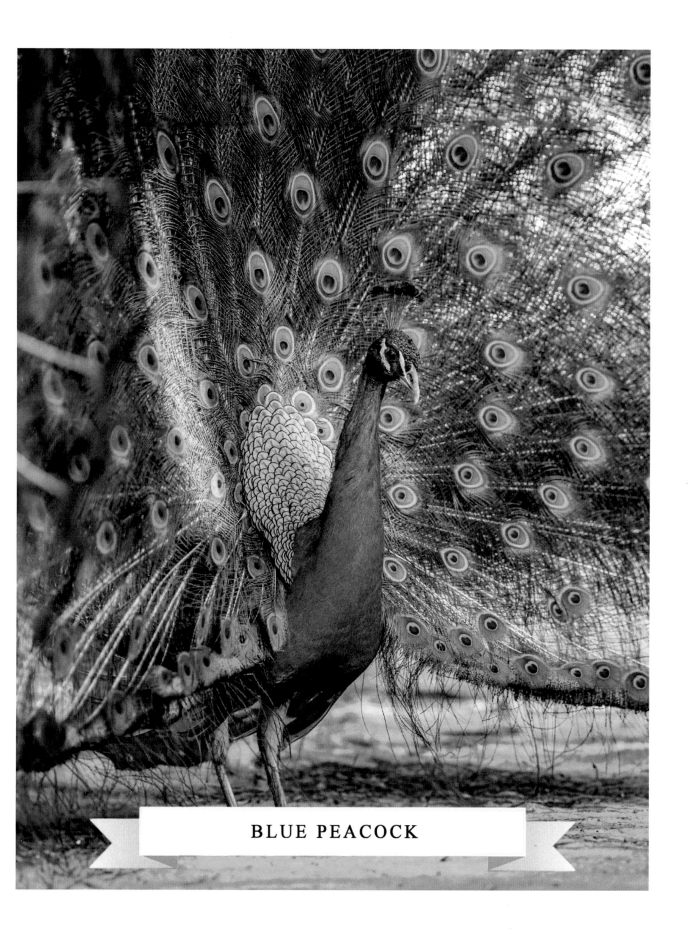

BLUE PEACOCK

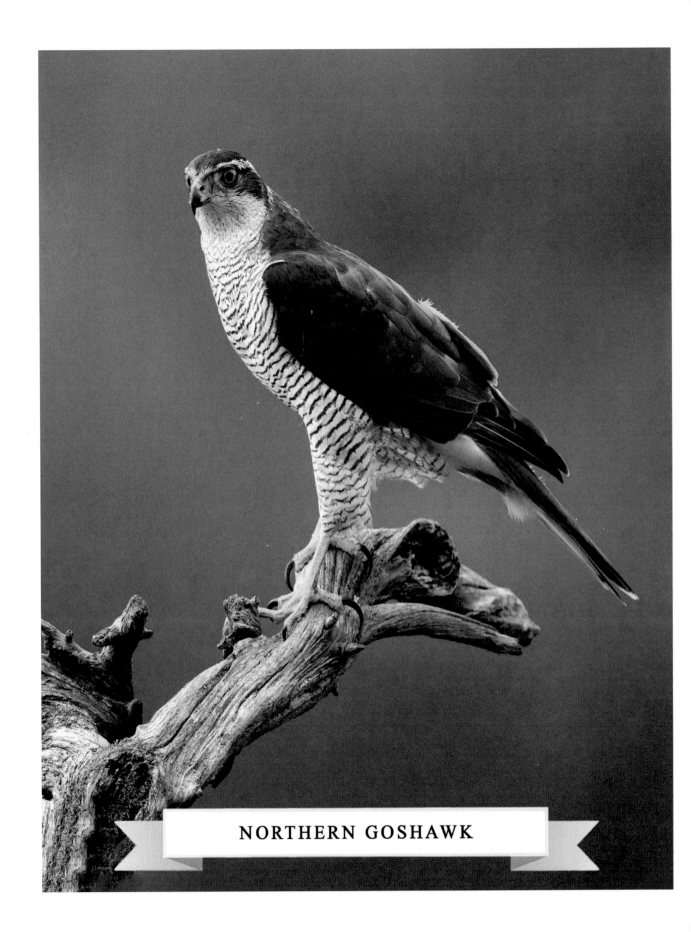

NORTHERN GOSHAWK

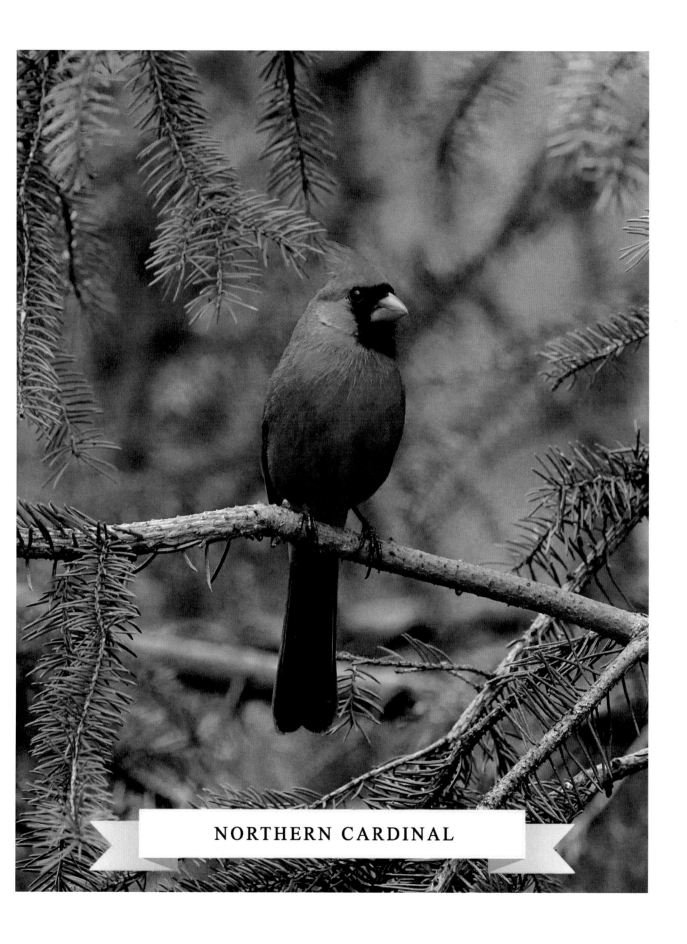

NORTHERN CARDINAL

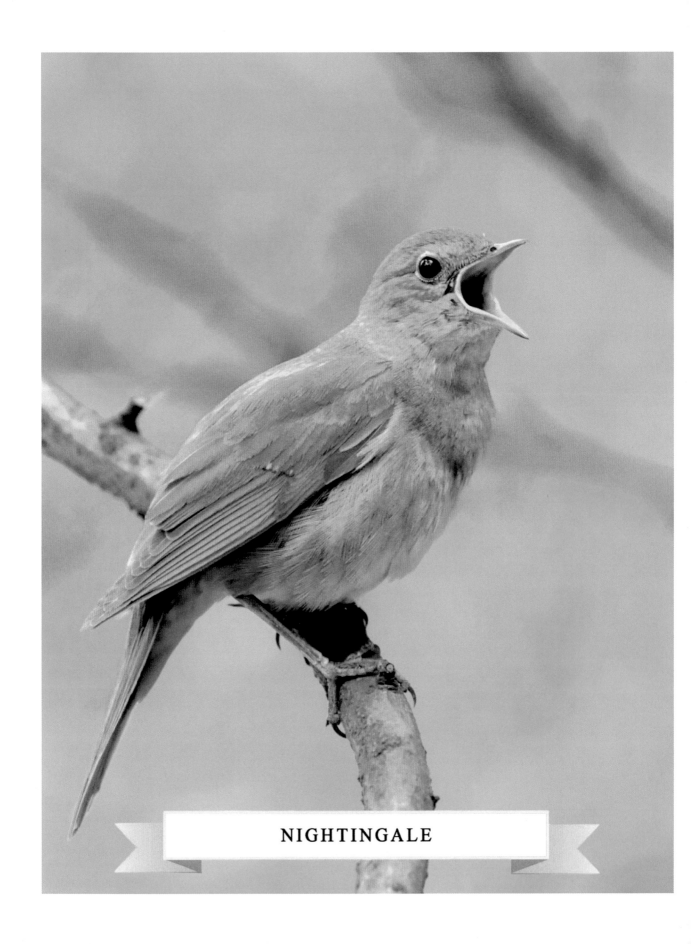

NIGHTINGALE

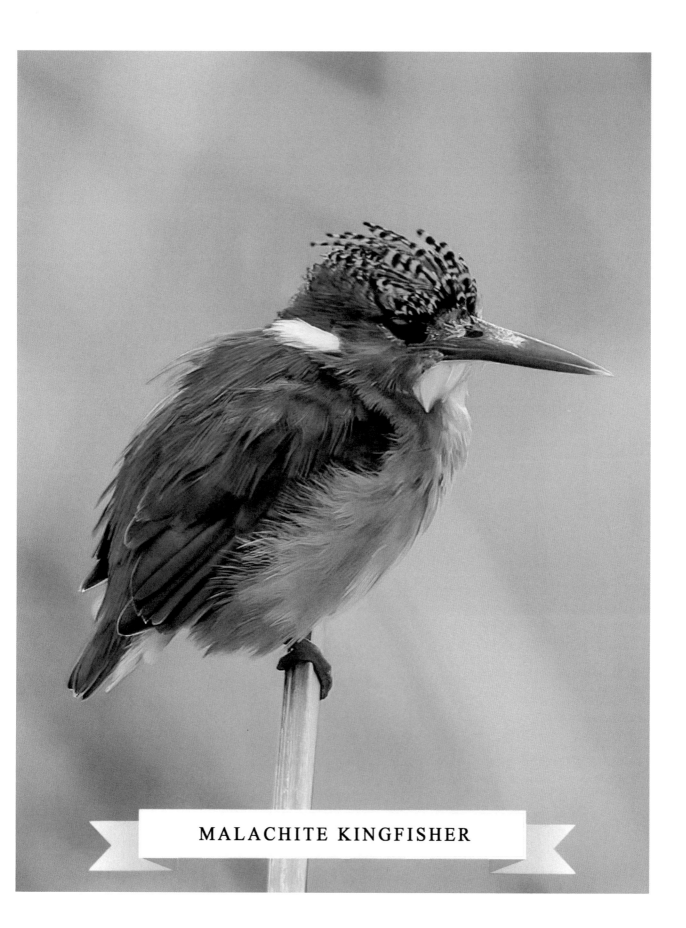

MALACHITE KINGFISHER

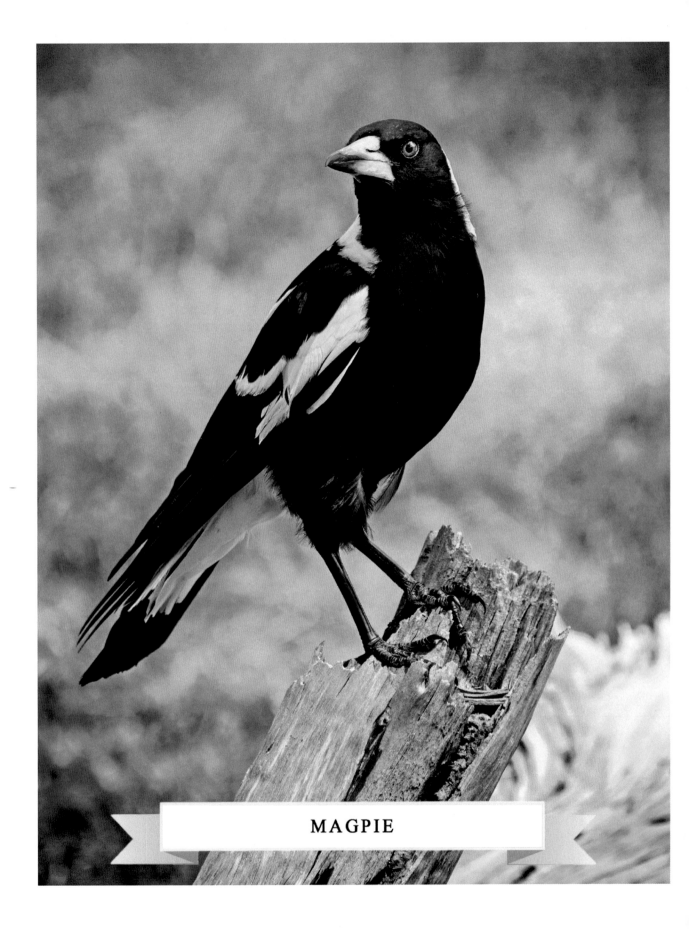

MAGPIE

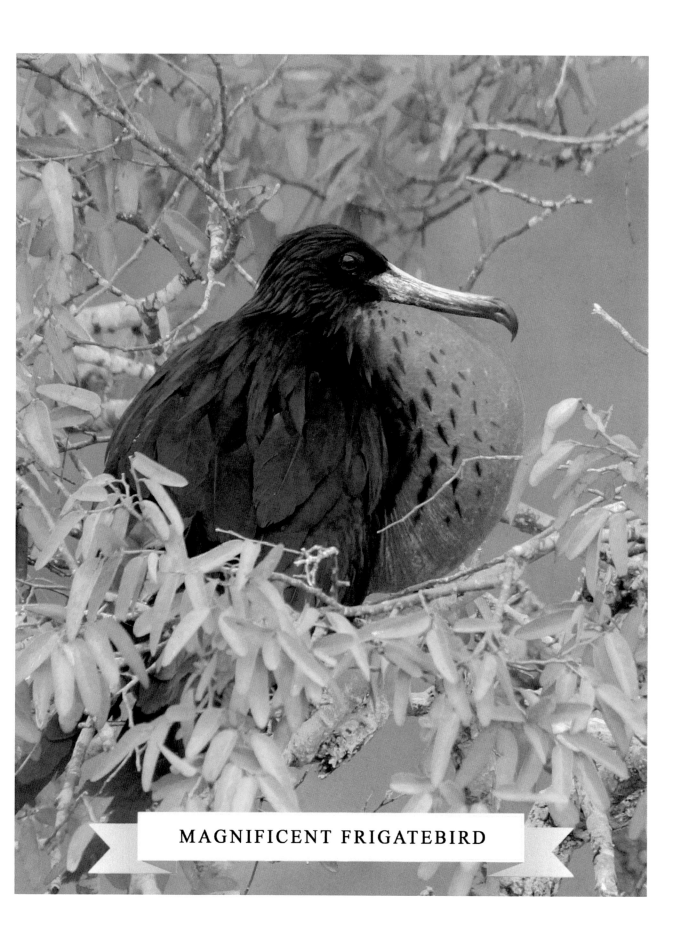

MAGNIFICENT FRIGATEBIRD

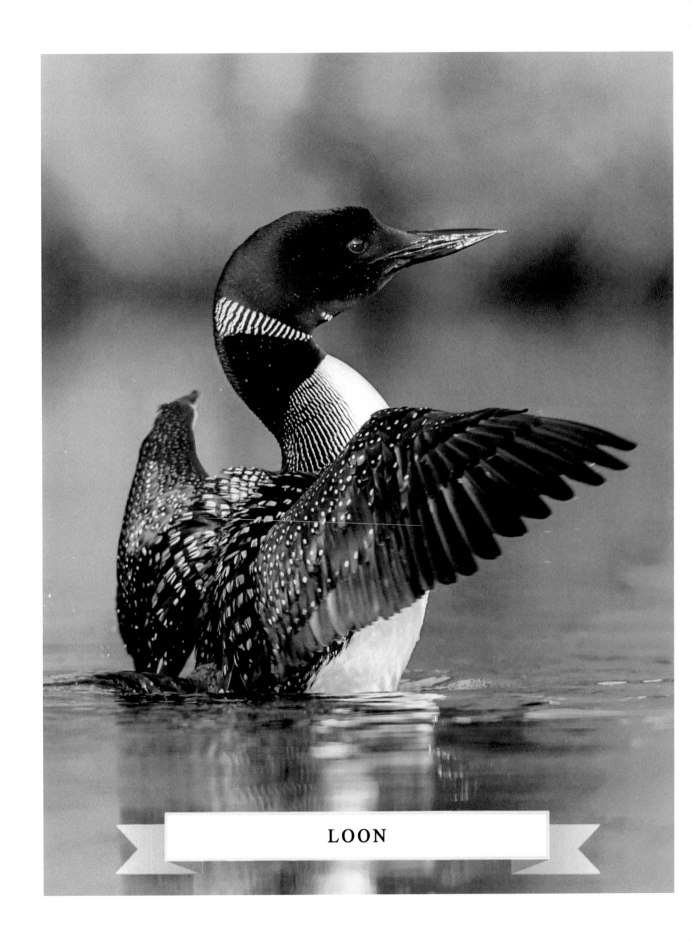

LOON

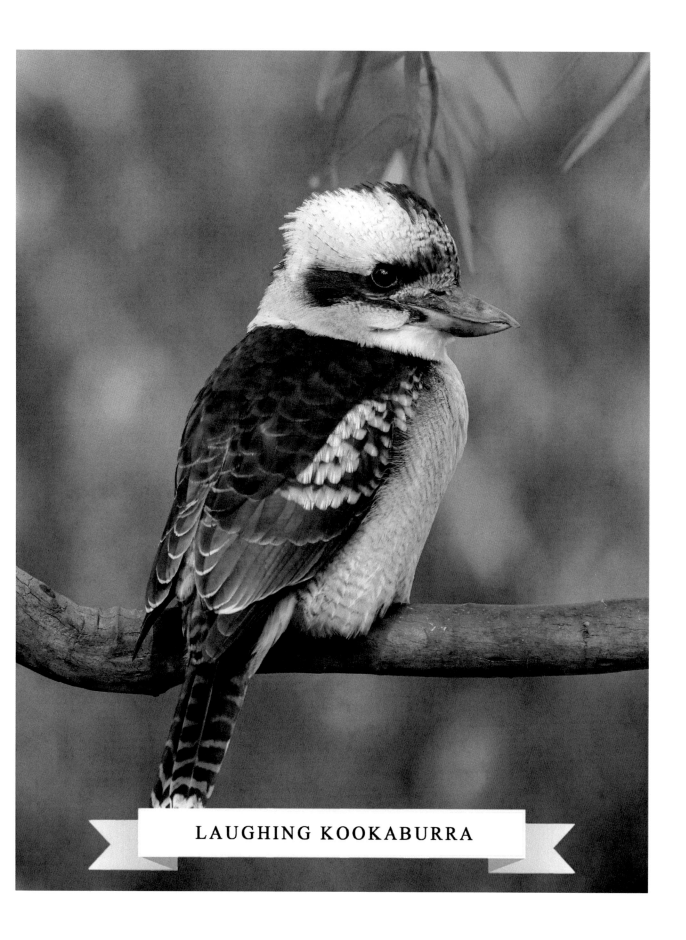

LAUGHING KOOKABURRA

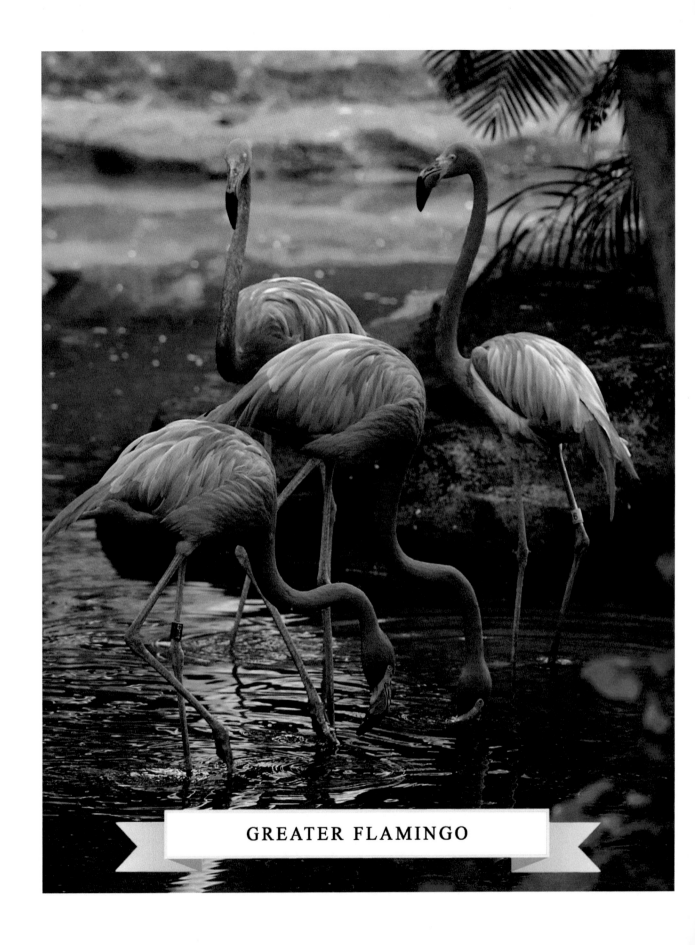

GREATER FLAMINGO

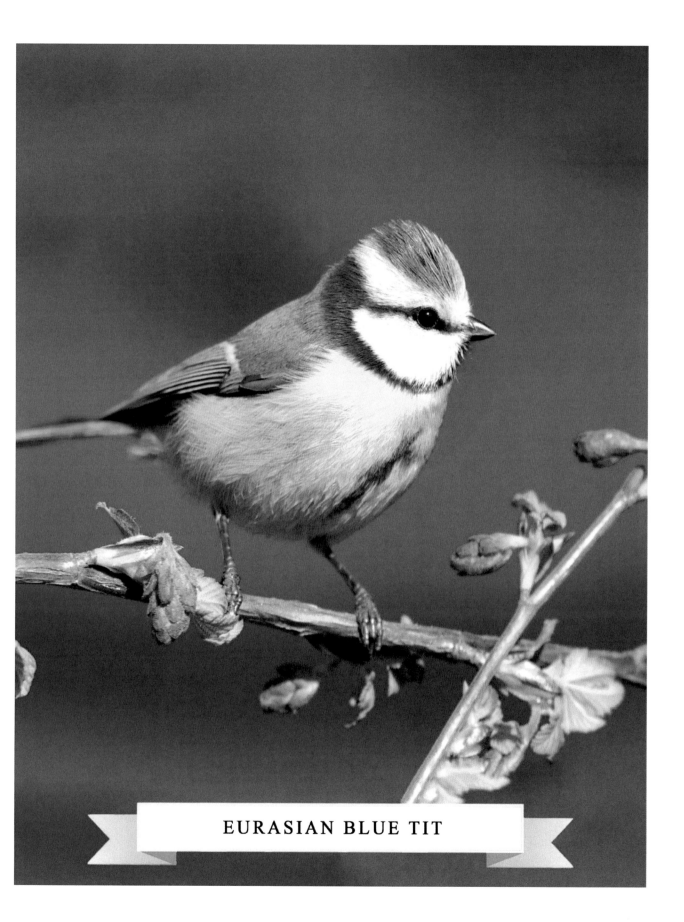

EURASIAN BLUE TIT

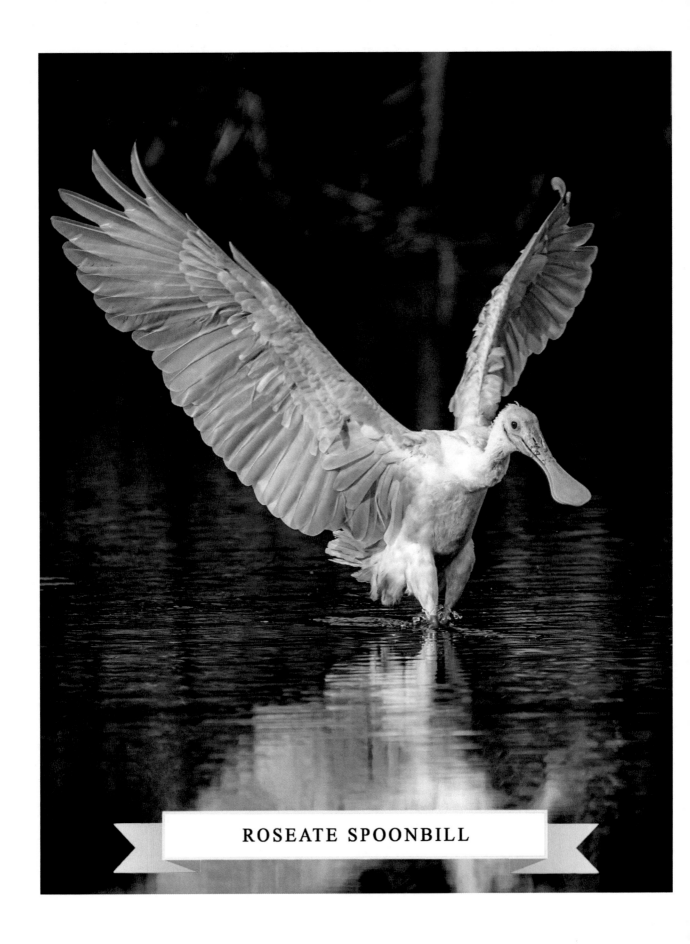

ROSEATE SPOONBILL

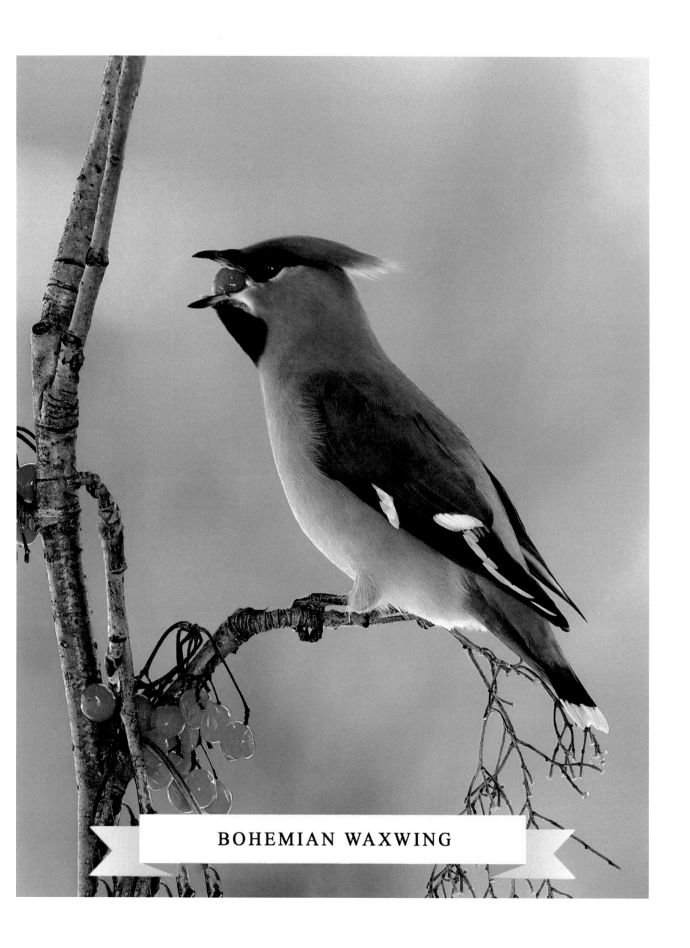

BOHEMIAN WAXWING

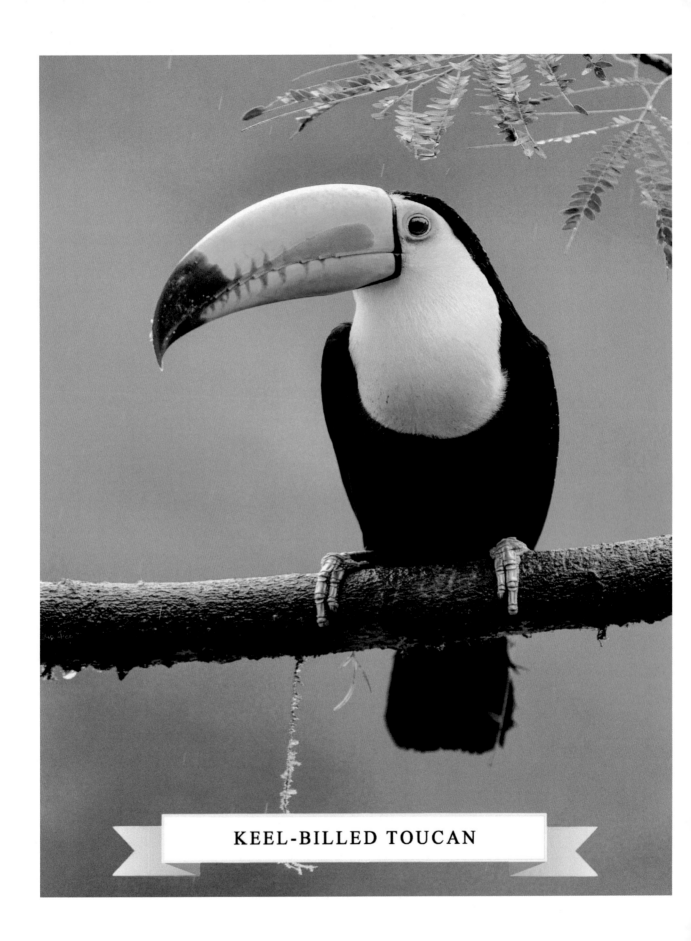

KEEL-BILLED TOUCAN

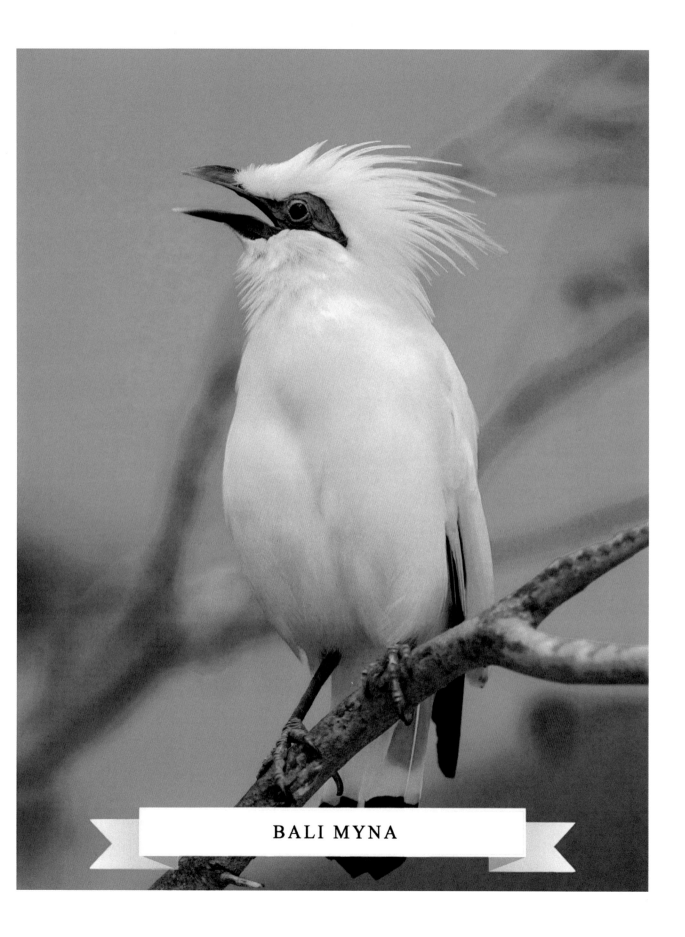

BALI MYNA

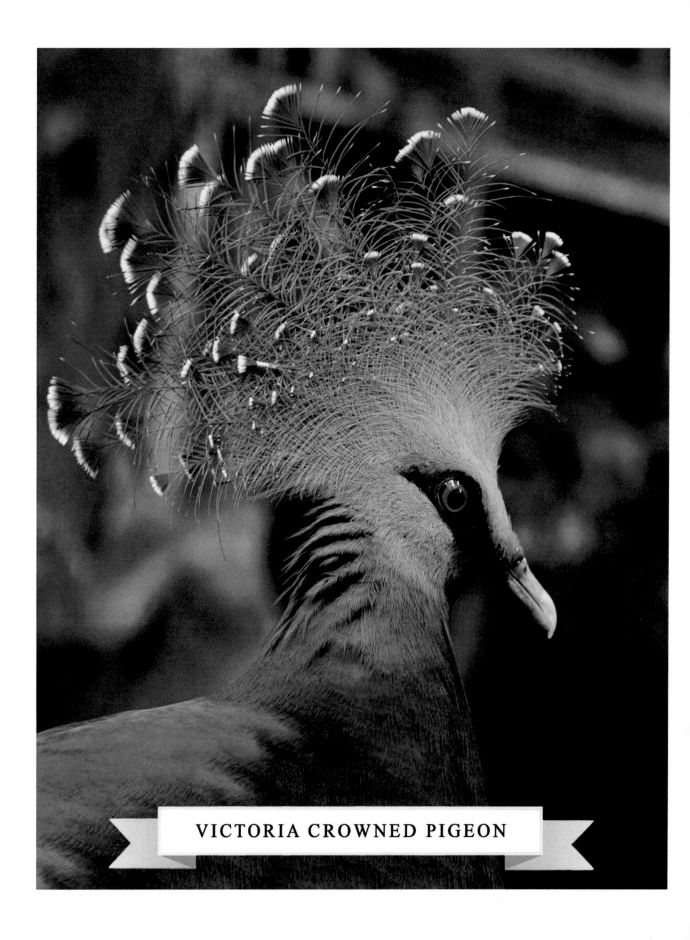

VICTORIA CROWNED PIGEON

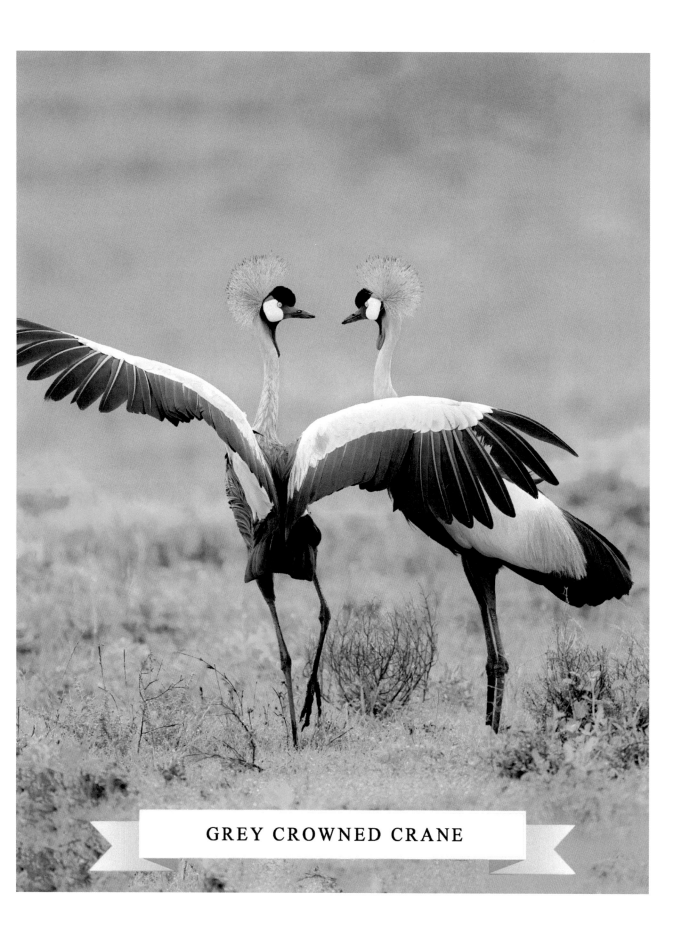

GREY CROWNED CRANE

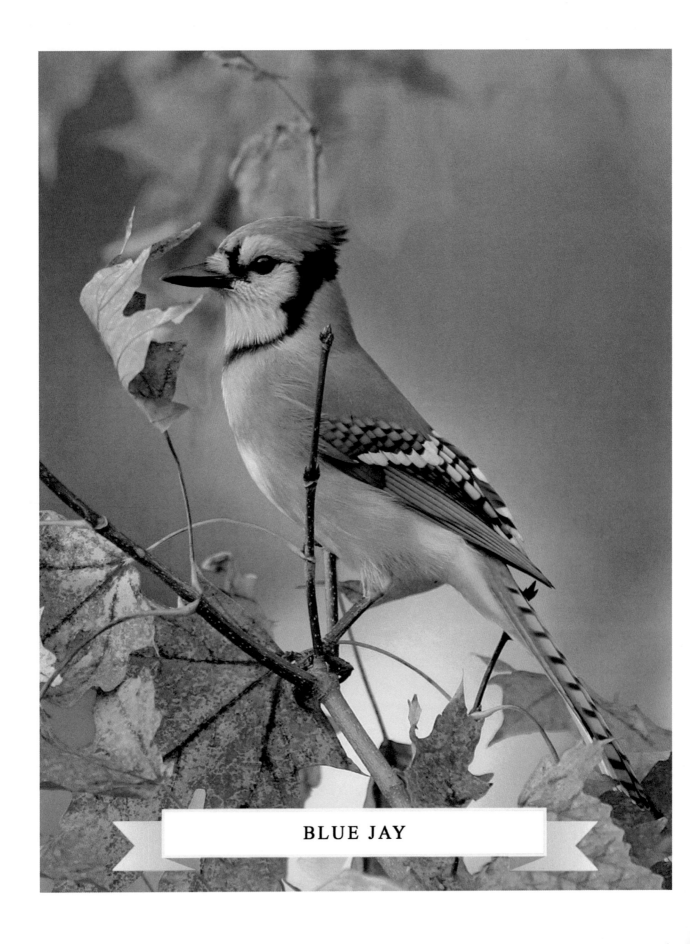

BLUE JAY

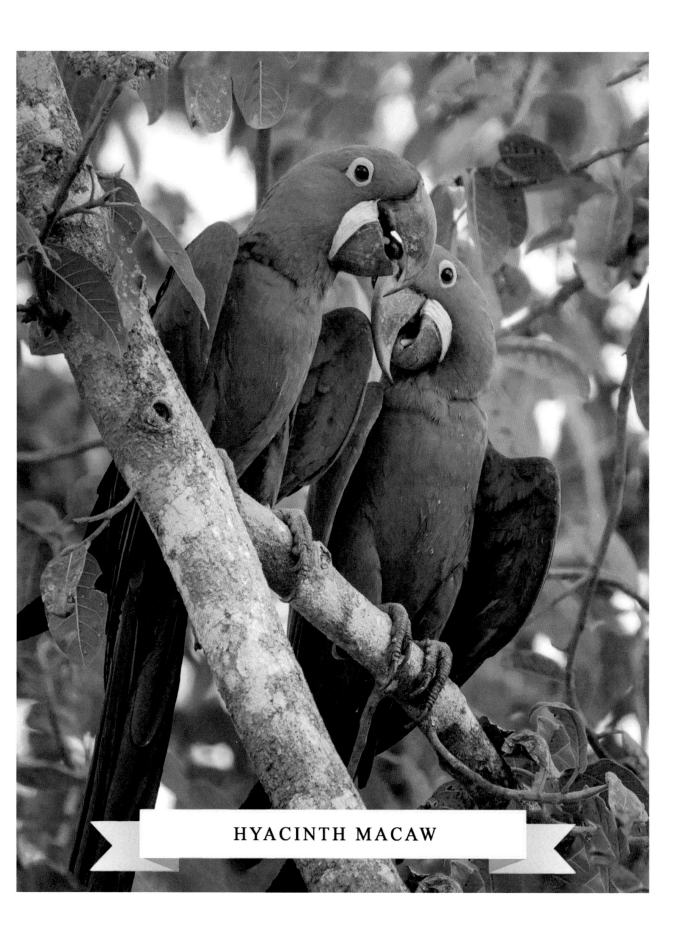

HYACINTH MACAW

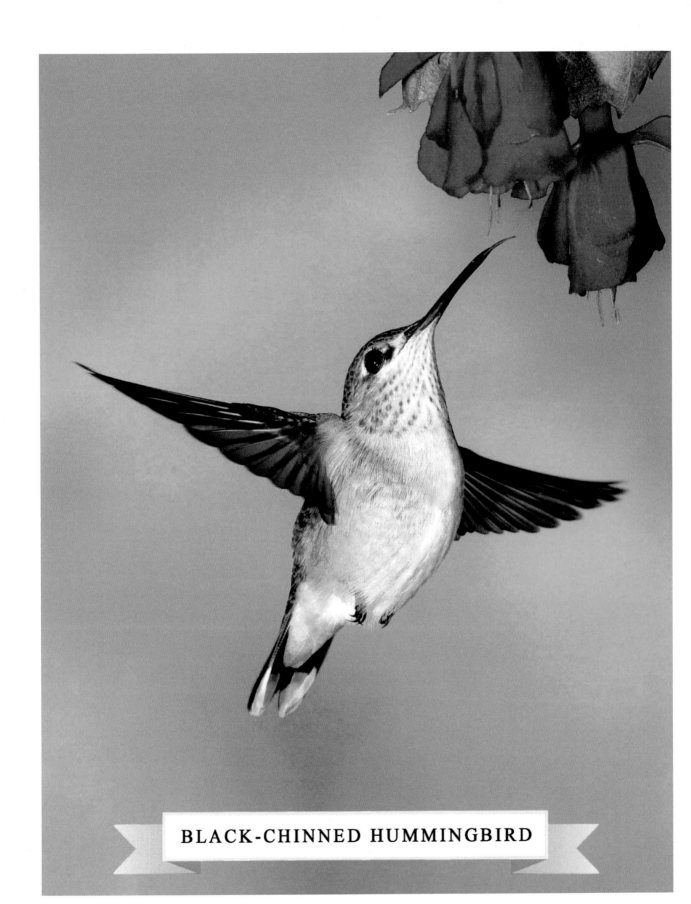

BLACK-CHINNED HUMMINGBIRD

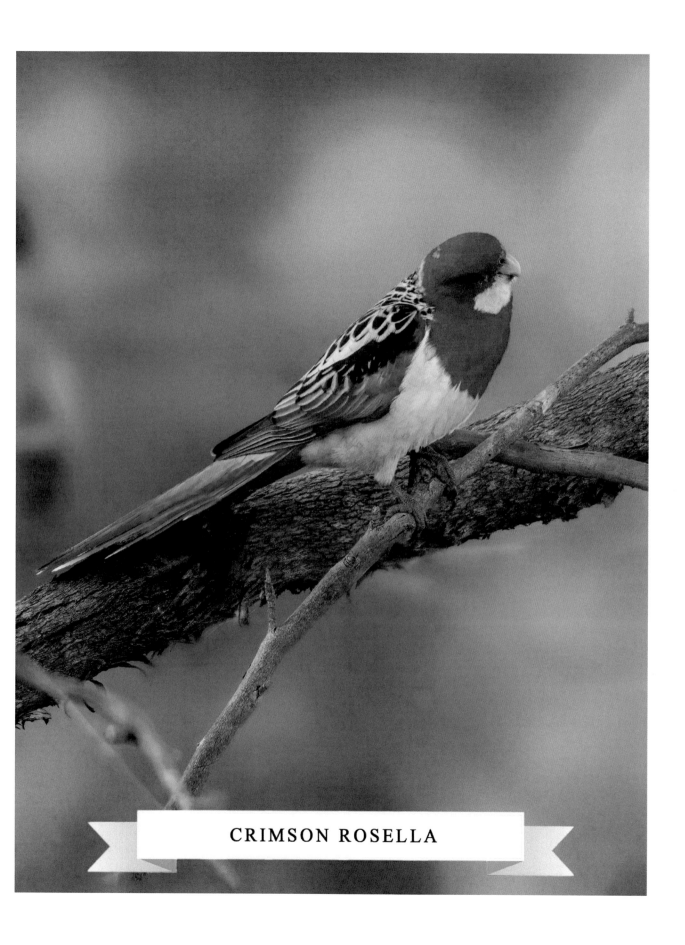

CRIMSON ROSELLA

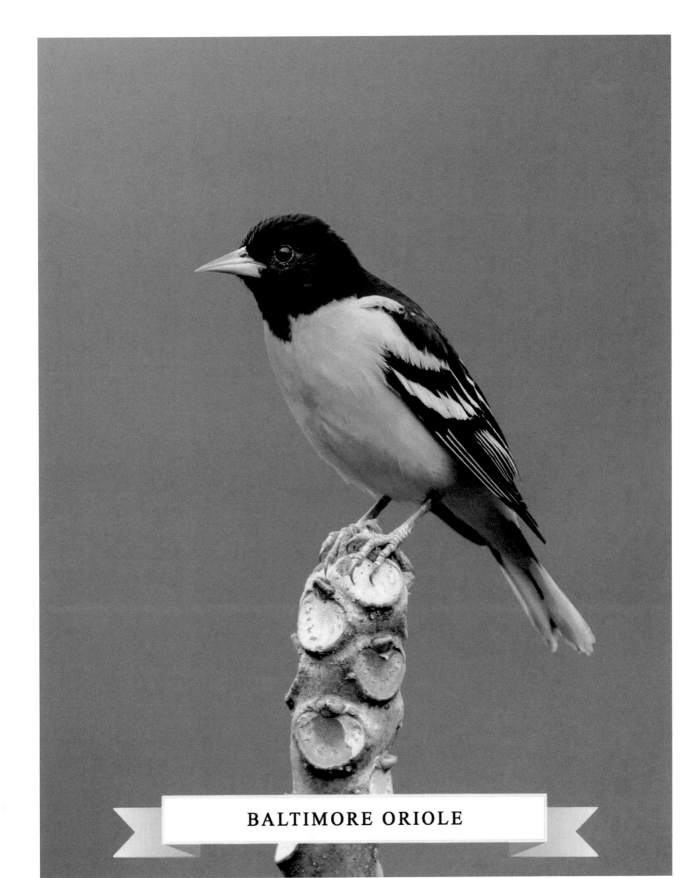

BALTIMORE ORIOLE

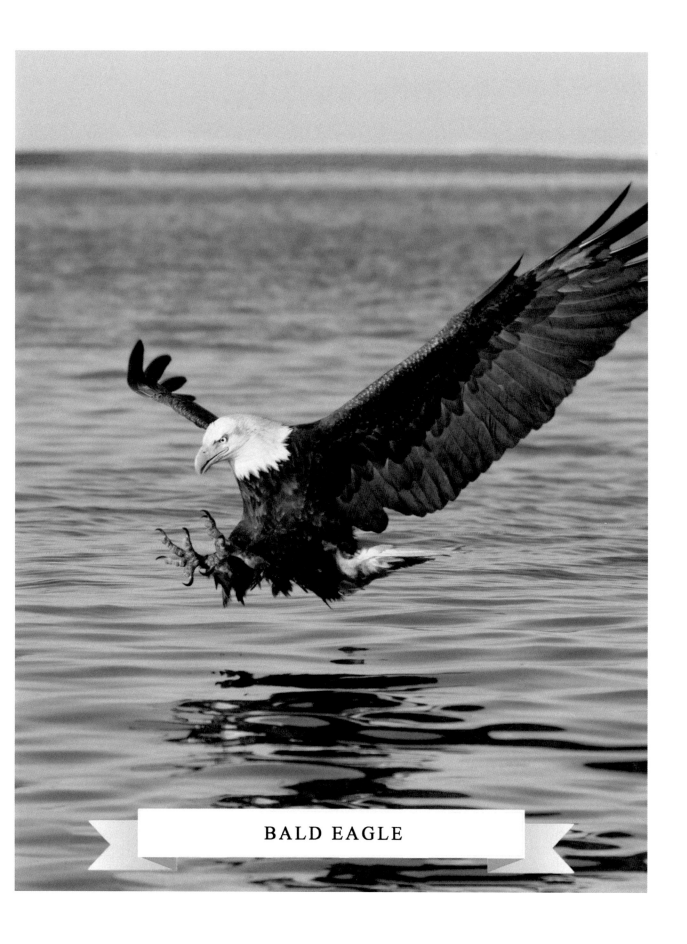

BALD EAGLE

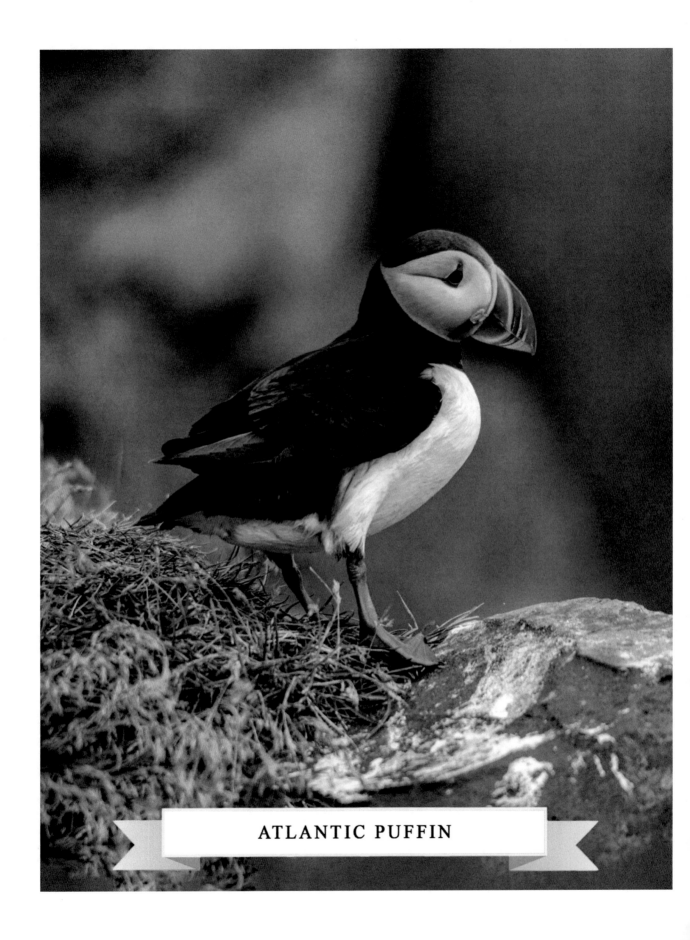

ATLANTIC PUFFIN

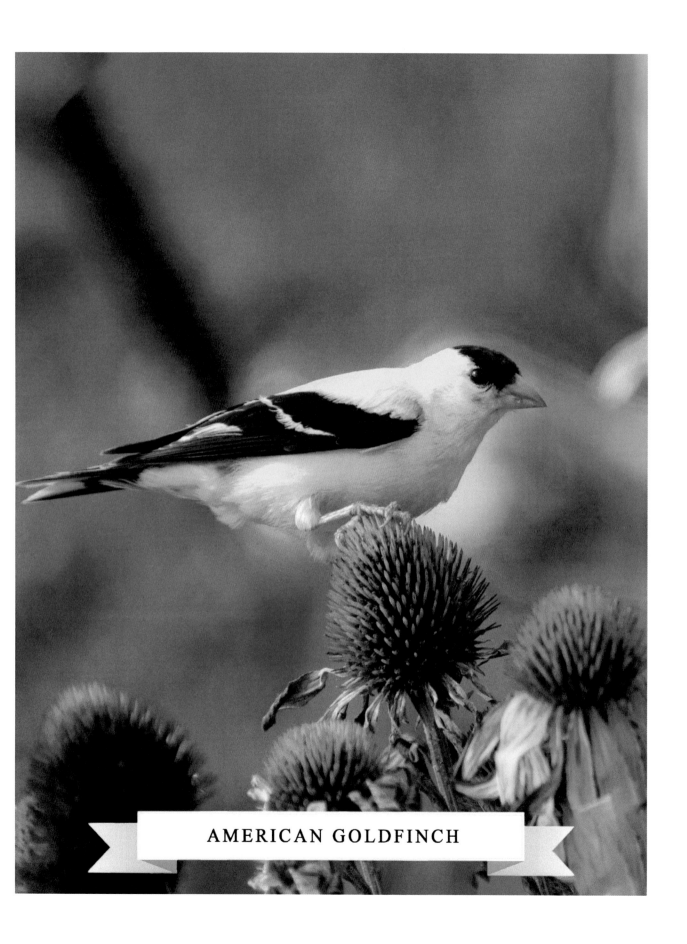

AMERICAN GOLDFINCH

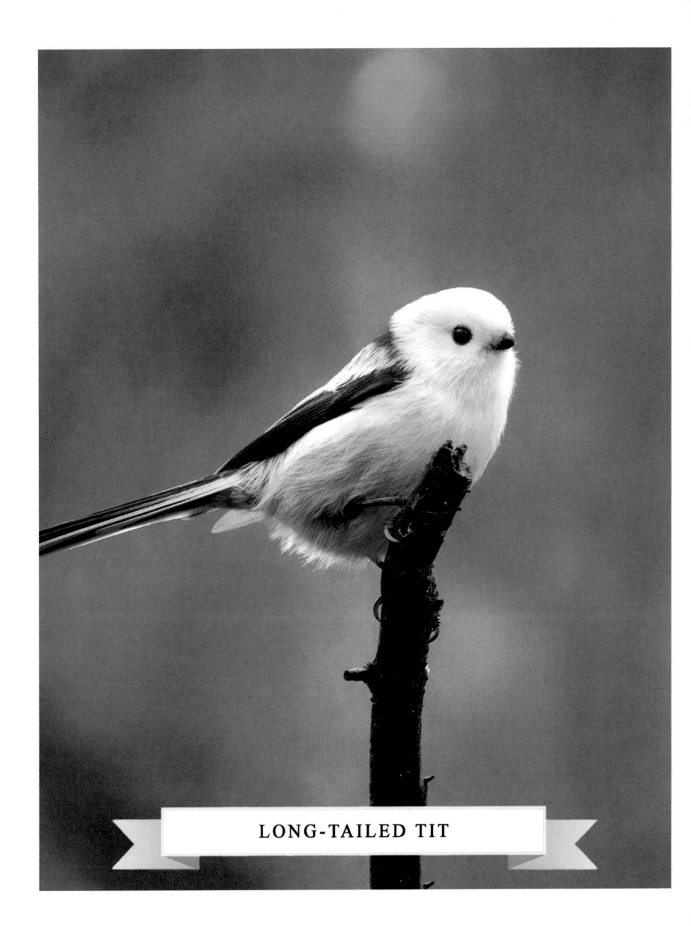

LONG-TAILED TIT

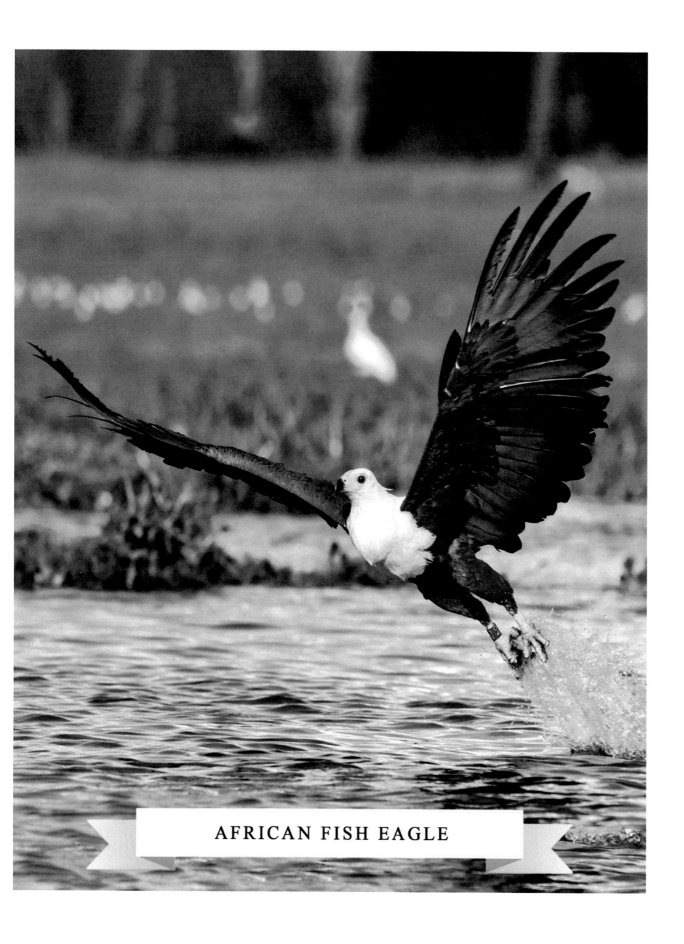

AFRICAN FISH EAGLE

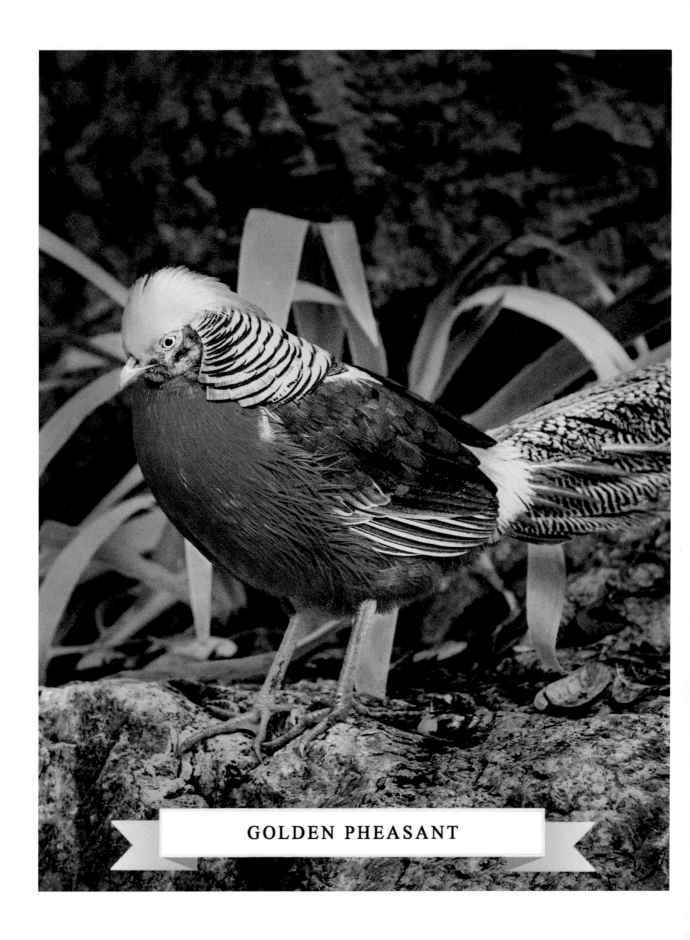

GOLDEN PHEASANT

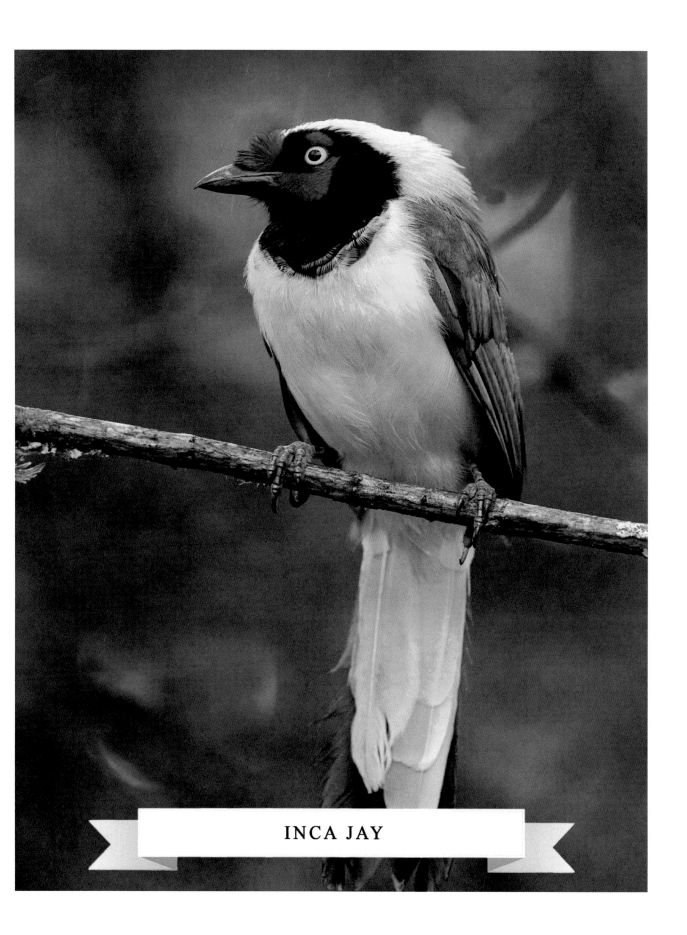

INCA JAY

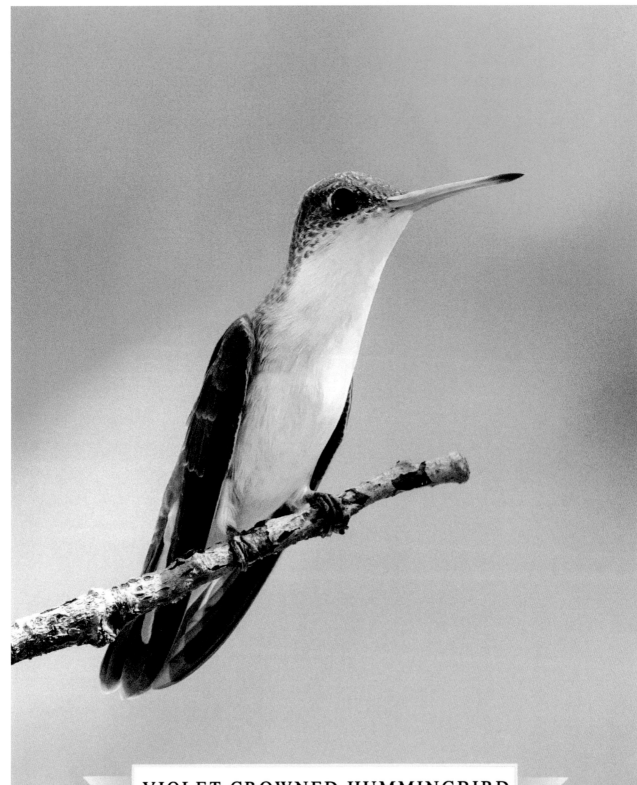

VIOLET-CROWNED HUMMINGBIRD

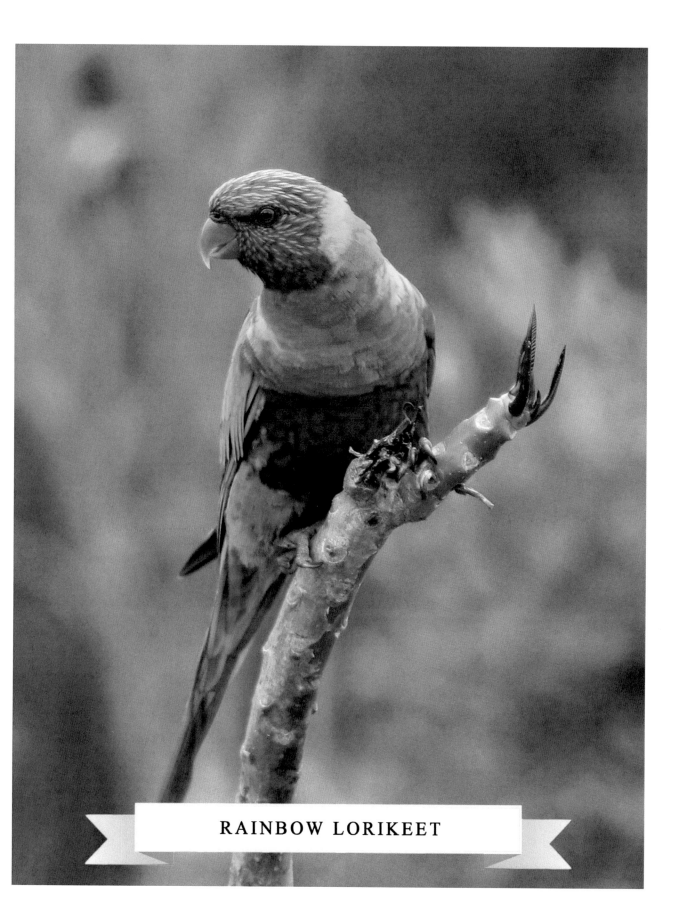

RAINBOW LORIKEET

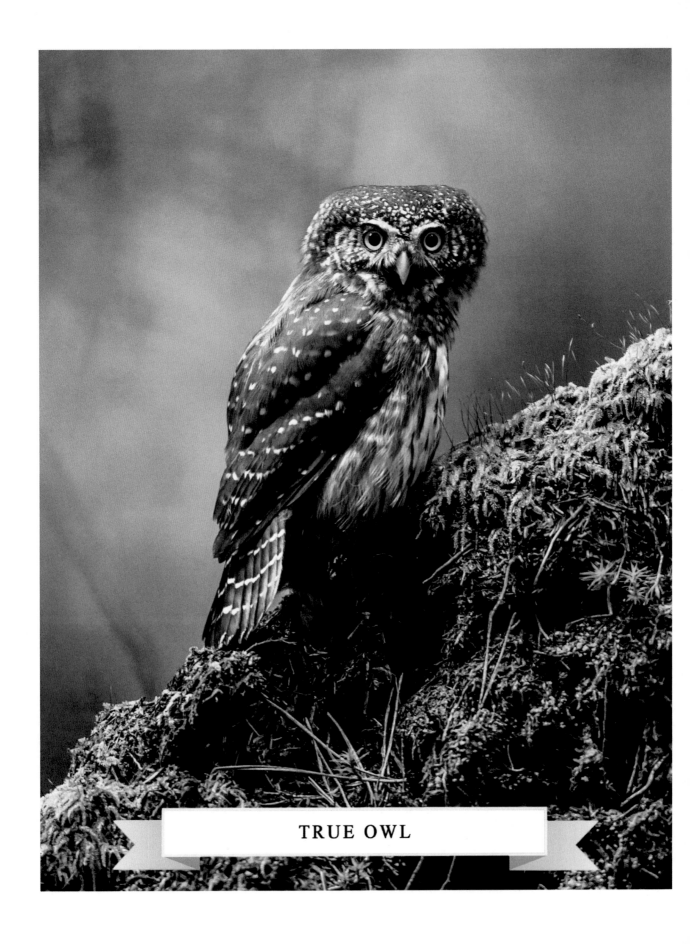

TRUE OWL

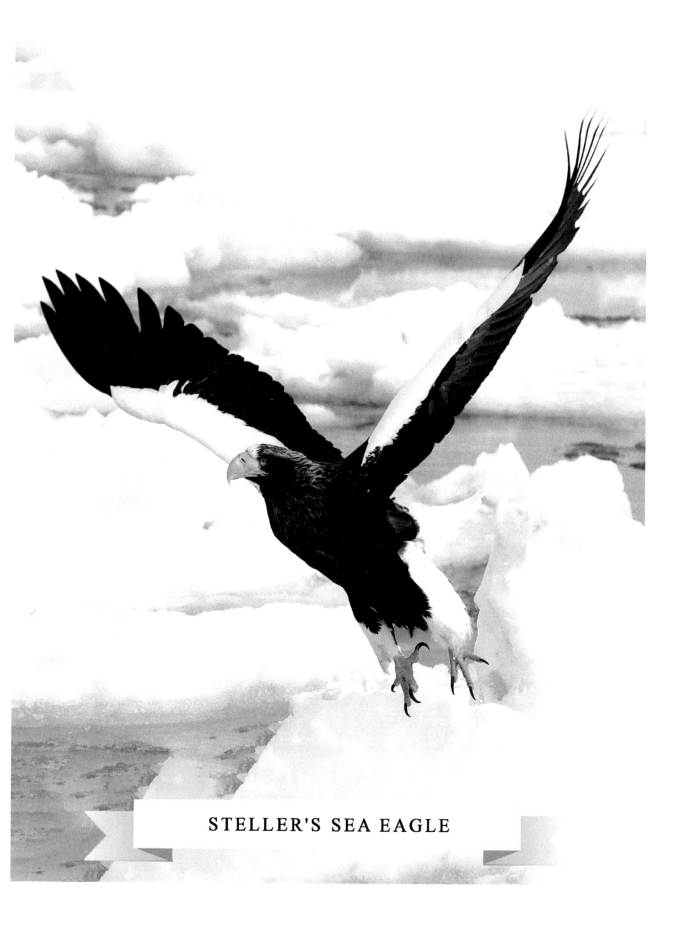

STELLER'S SEA EAGLE

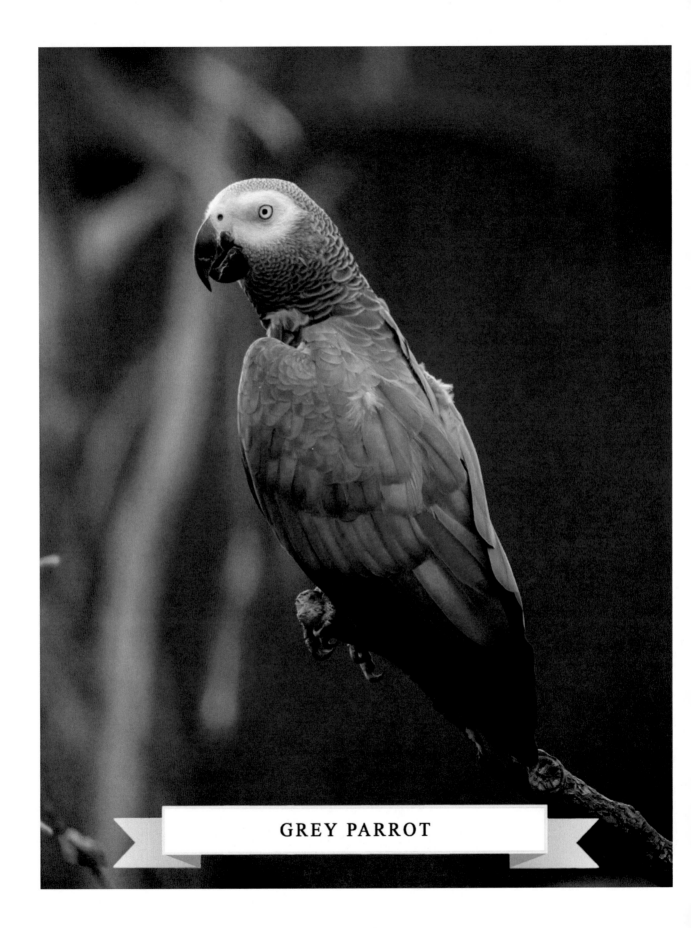

GREY PARROT

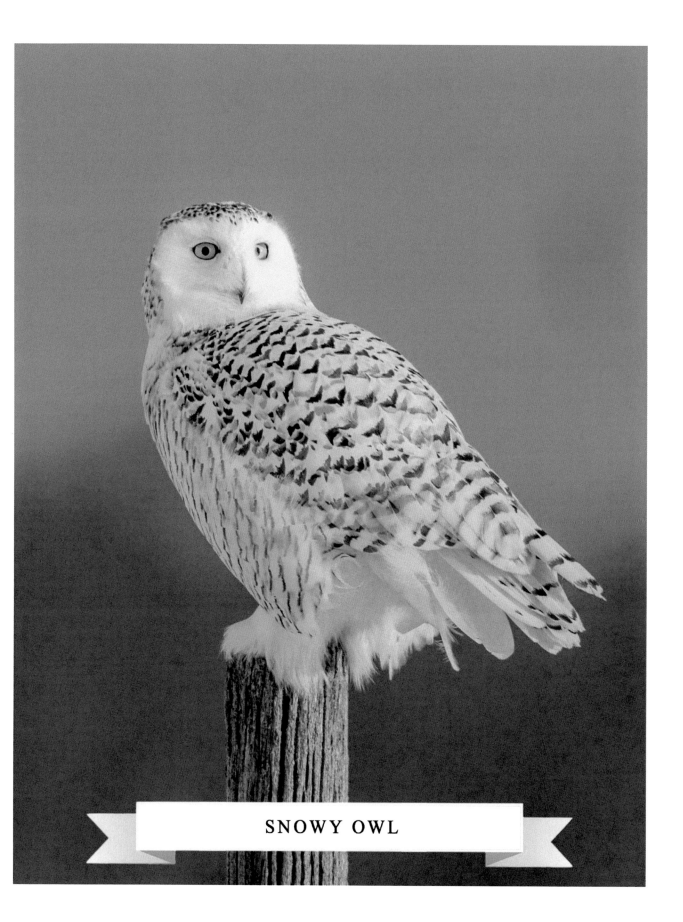

SNOWY OWL

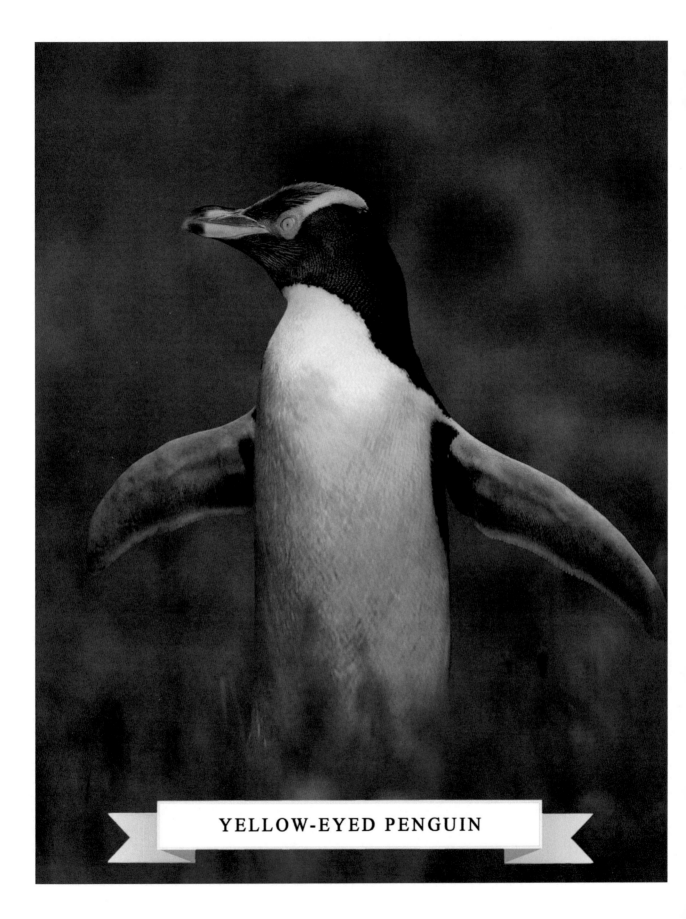

YELLOW-EYED PENGUIN

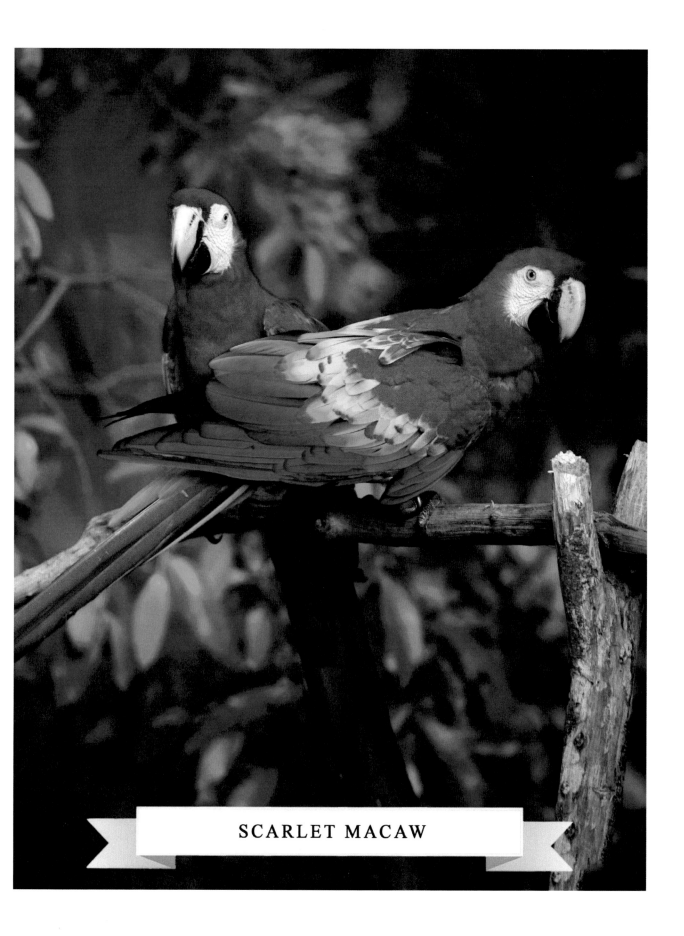

SCARLET MACAW

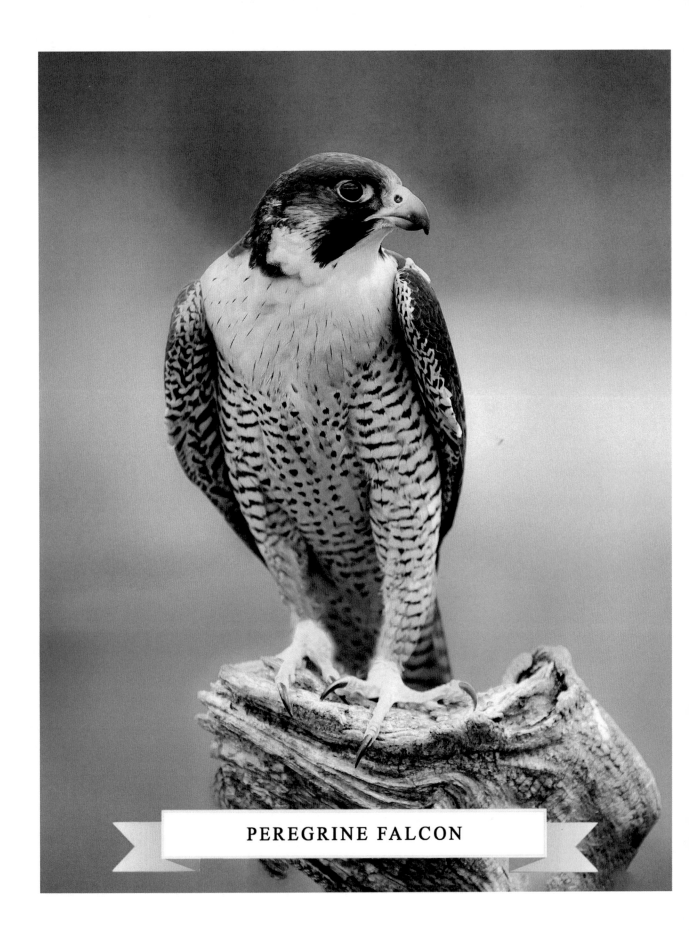

PEREGRINE FALCON

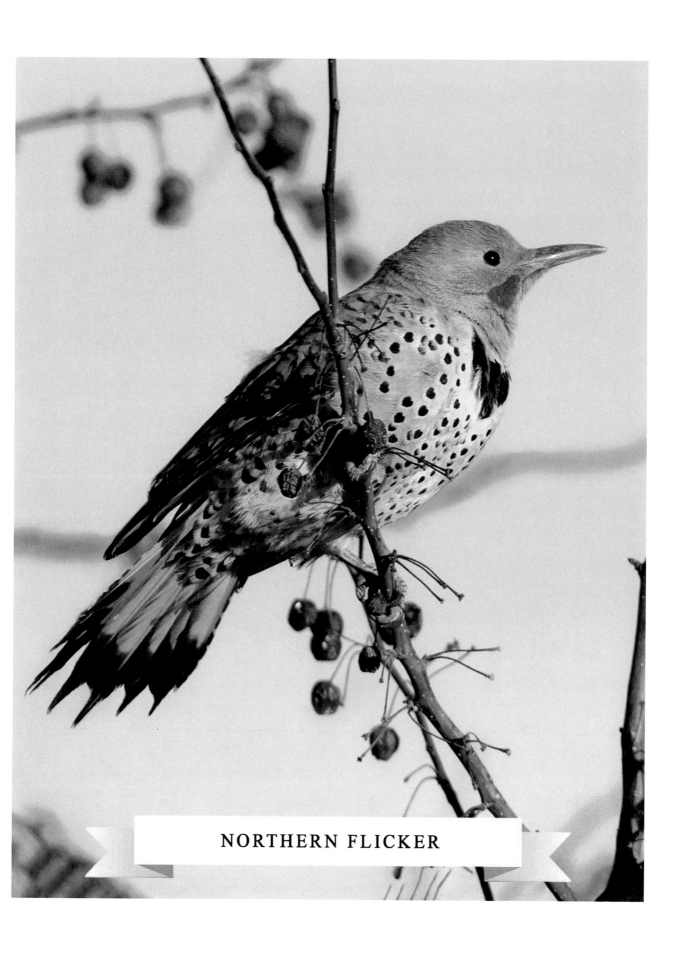

NORTHERN FLICKER

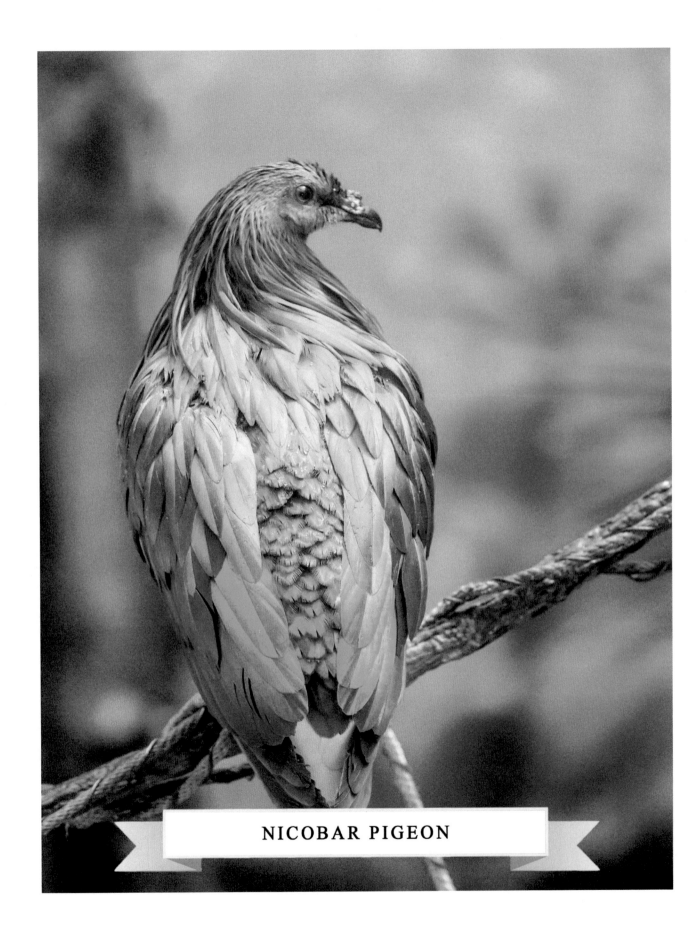

NICOBAR PIGEON

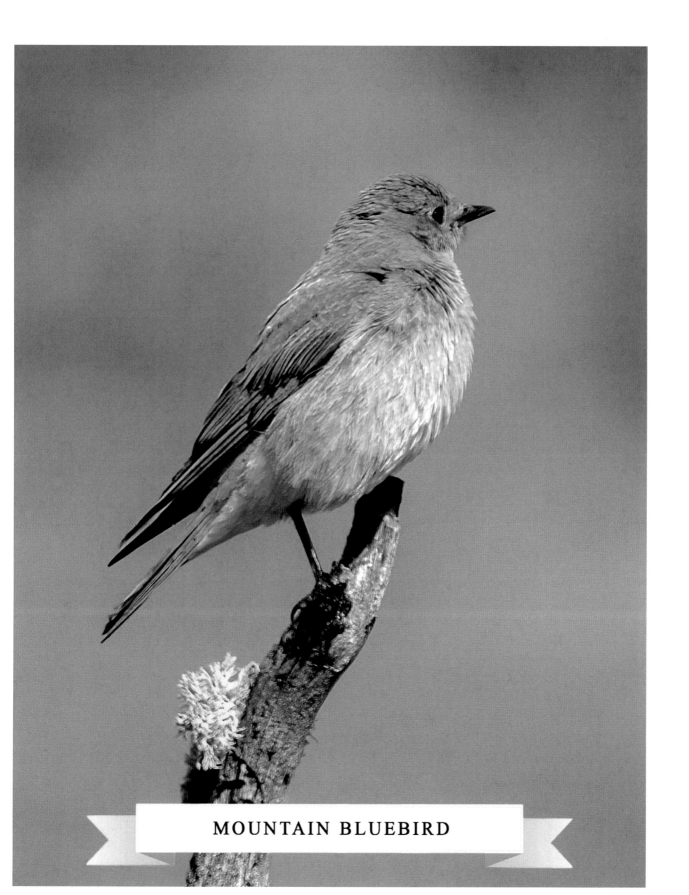

MOUNTAIN BLUEBIRD

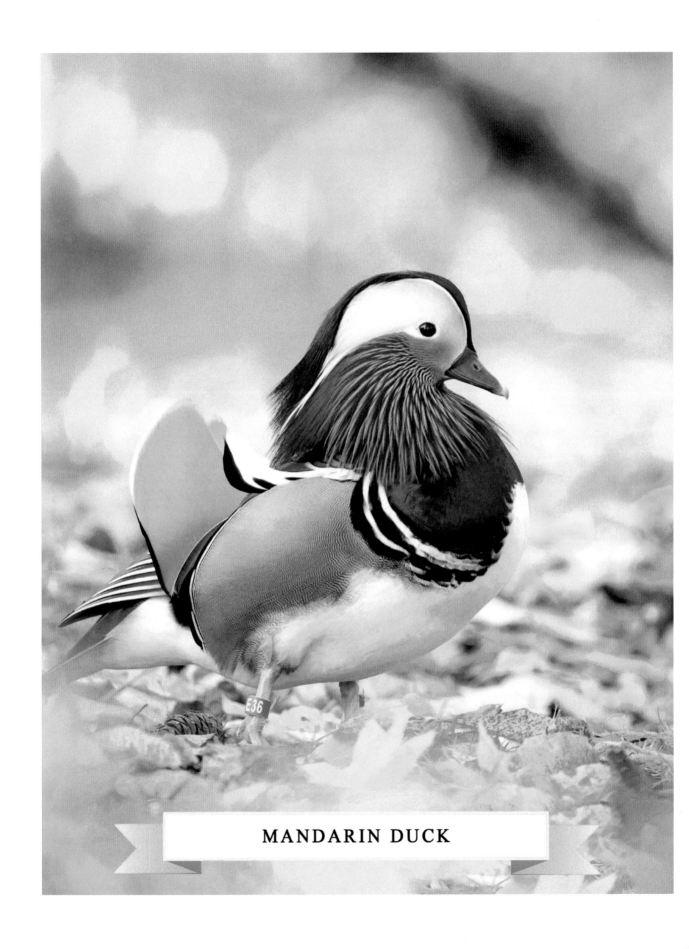

MANDARIN DUCK

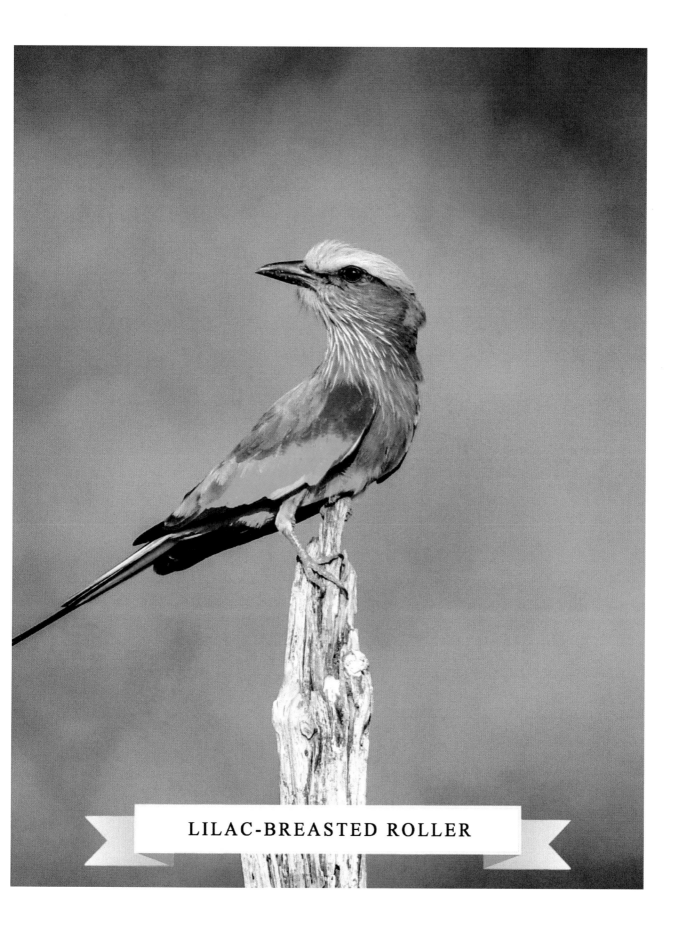

LILAC-BREASTED ROLLER

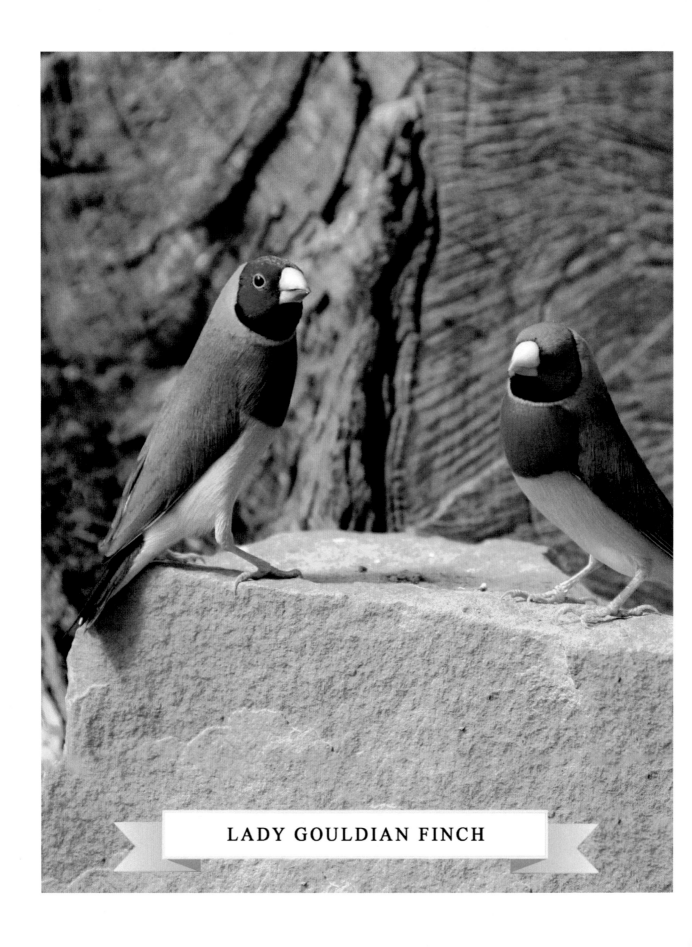

LADY GOULDIAN FINCH

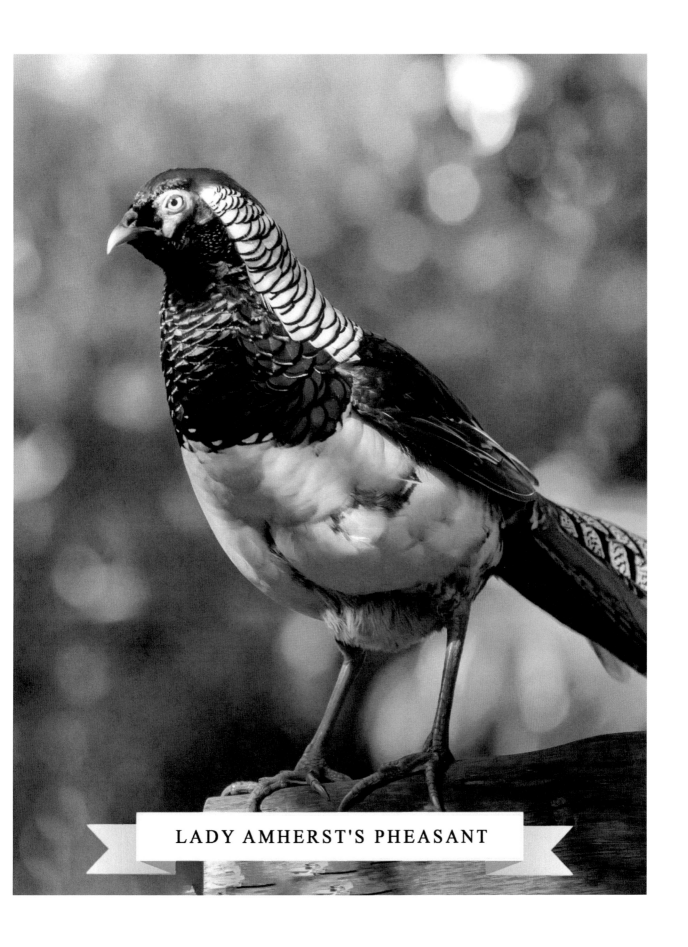

LADY AMHERST'S PHEASANT

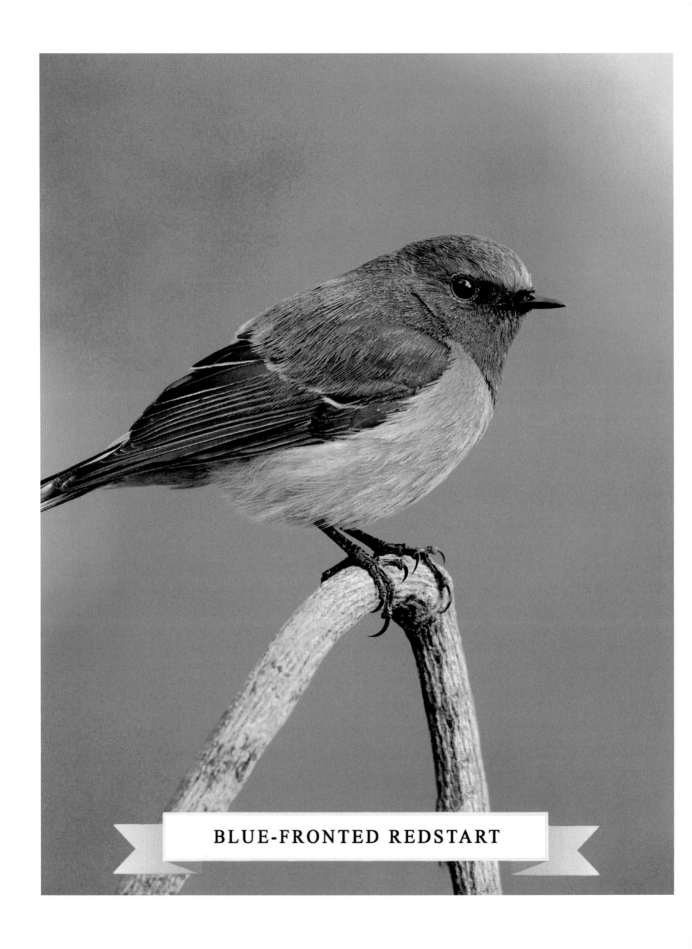

BLUE-FRONTED REDSTART

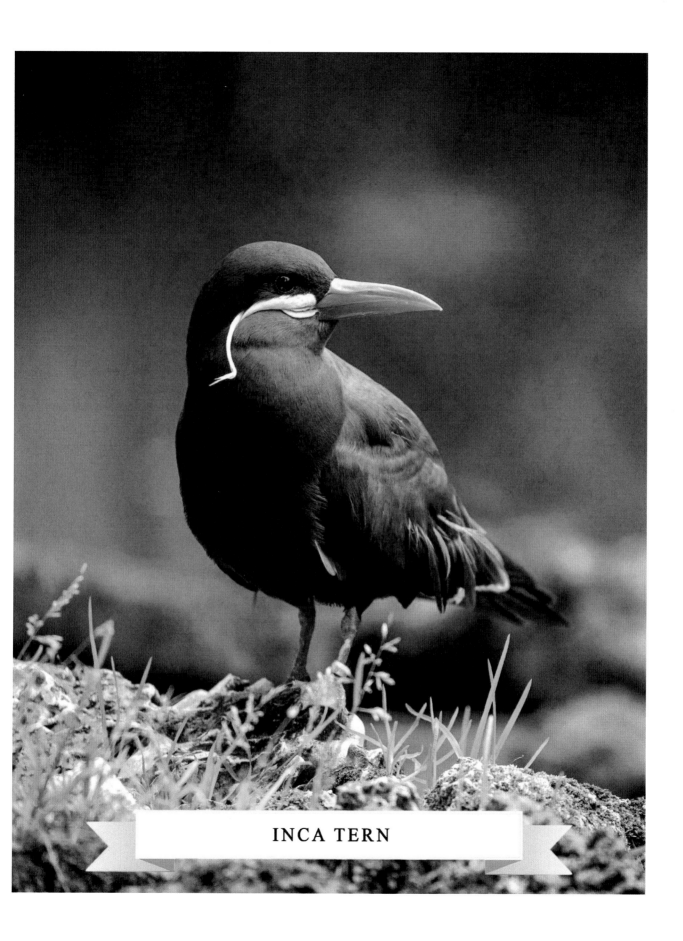

INCA TERN

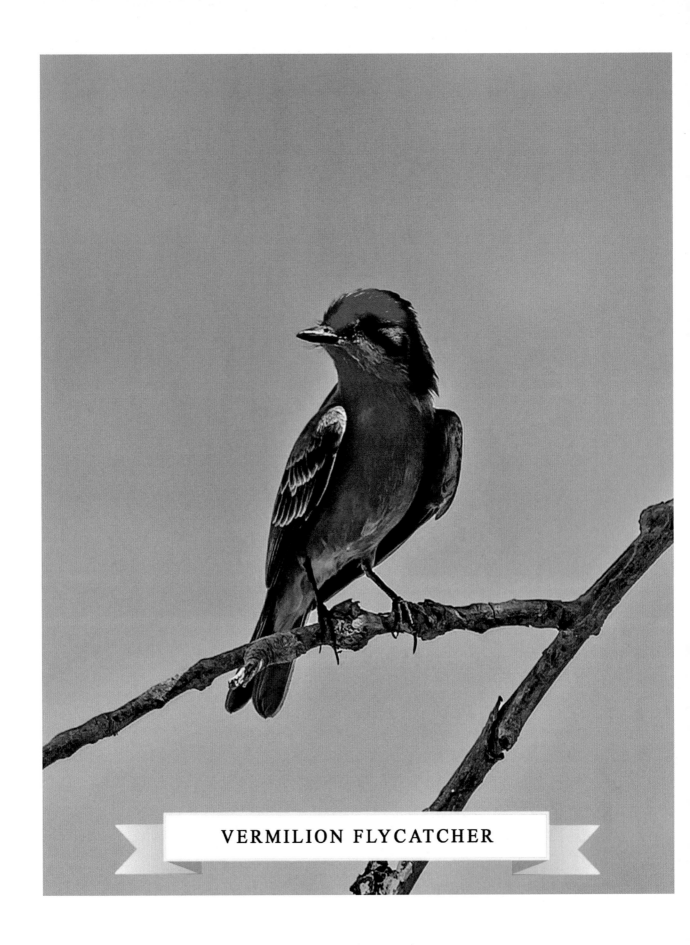

VERMILION FLYCATCHER

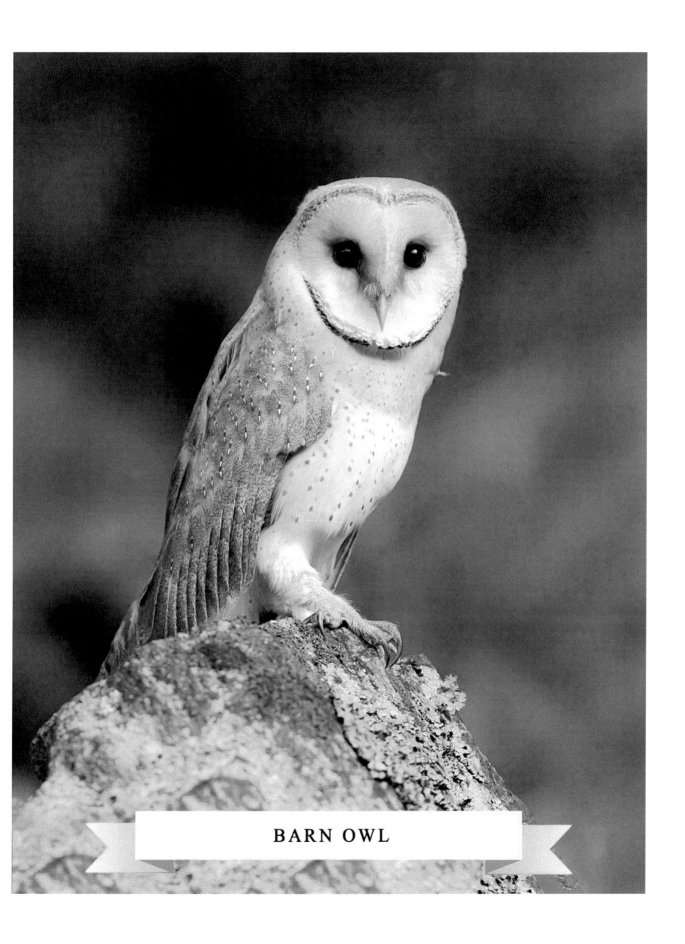

BARN OWL

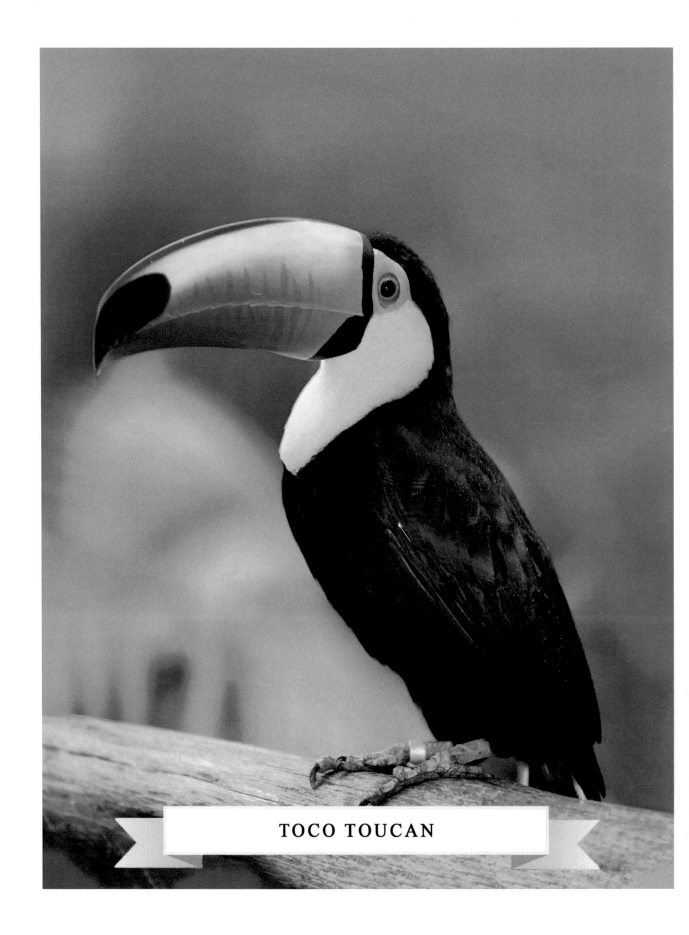

TOCO TOUCAN

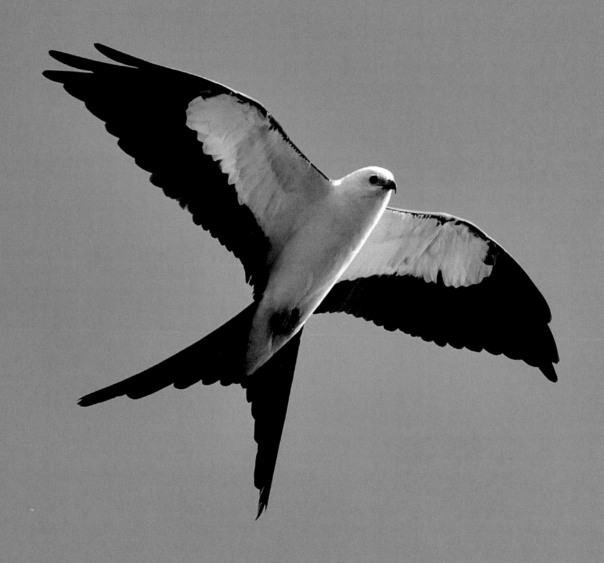

SWALLOW-TAILED KITE

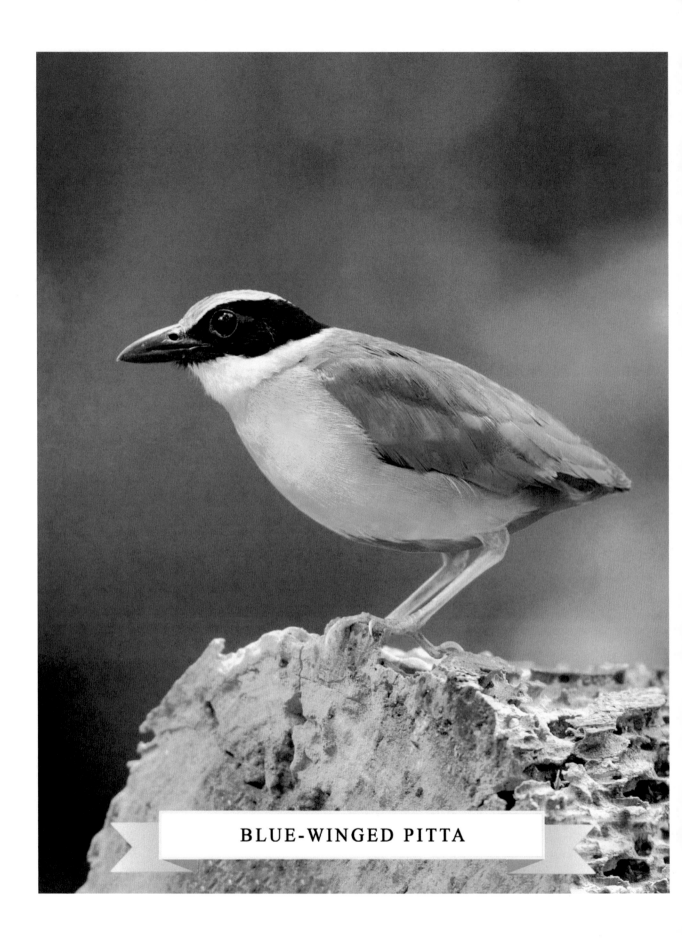

BLUE-WINGED PITTA

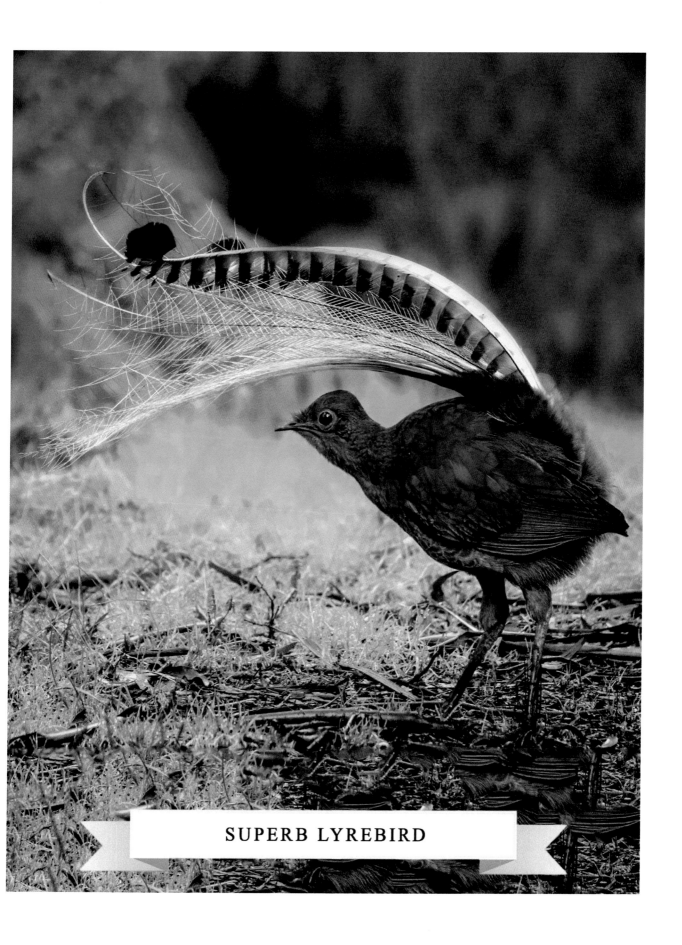

SUPERB LYREBIRD

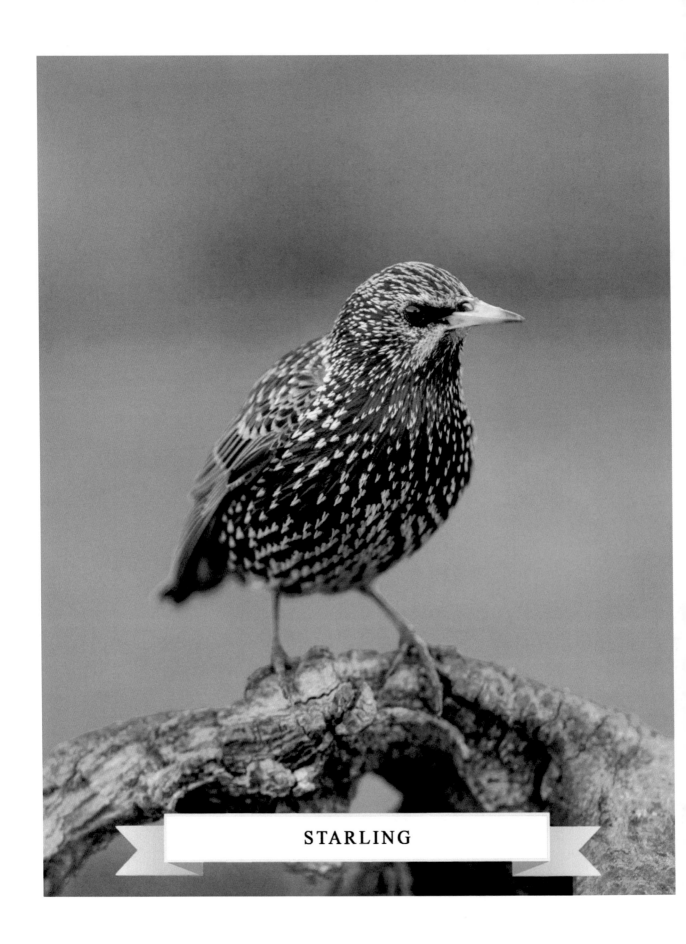

STARLING

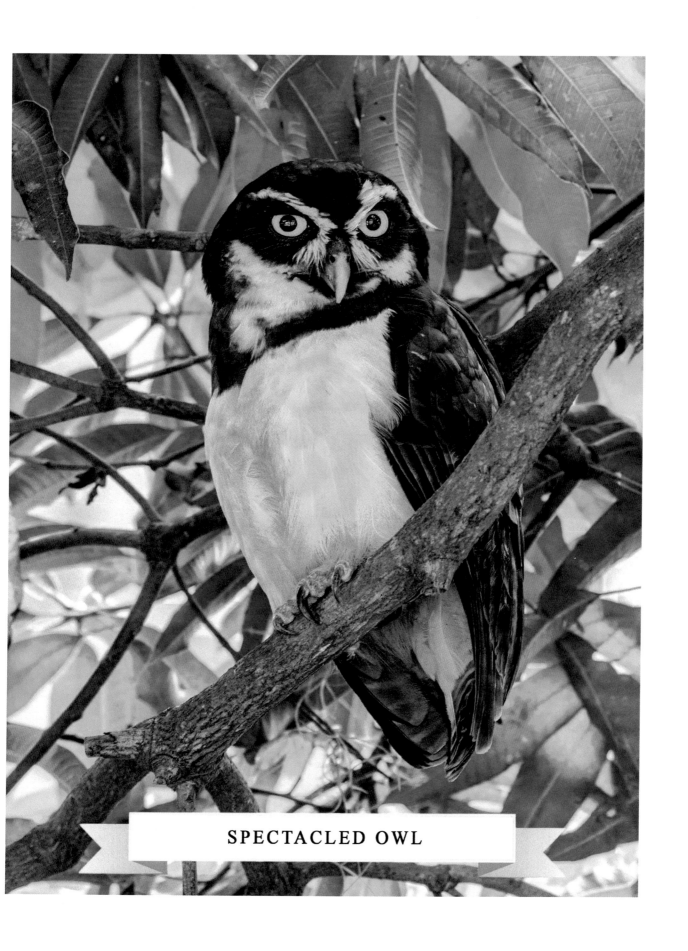

SPECTACLED OWL

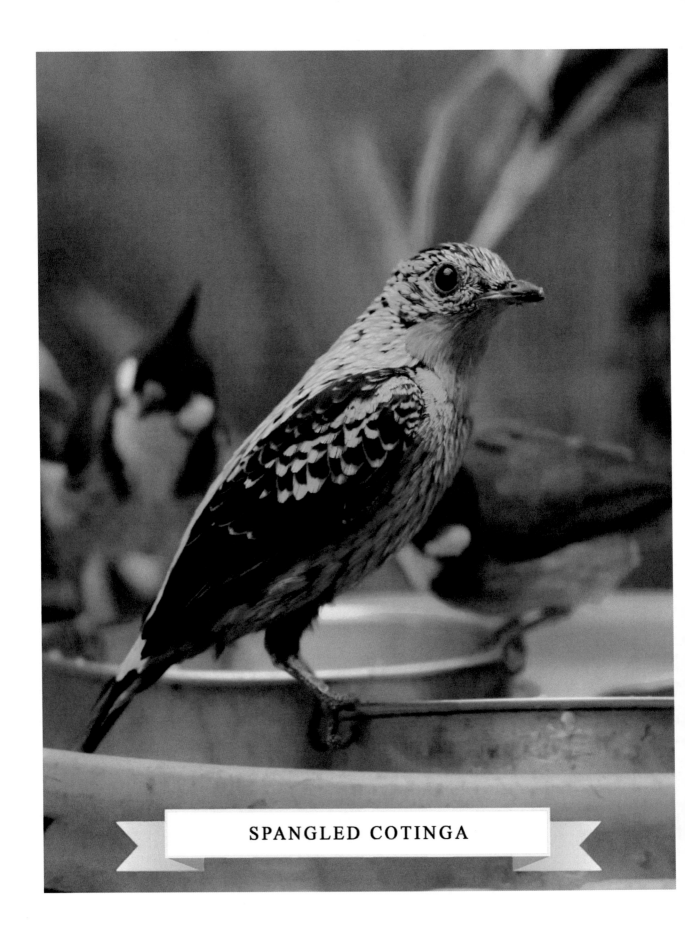

SPANGLED COTINGA

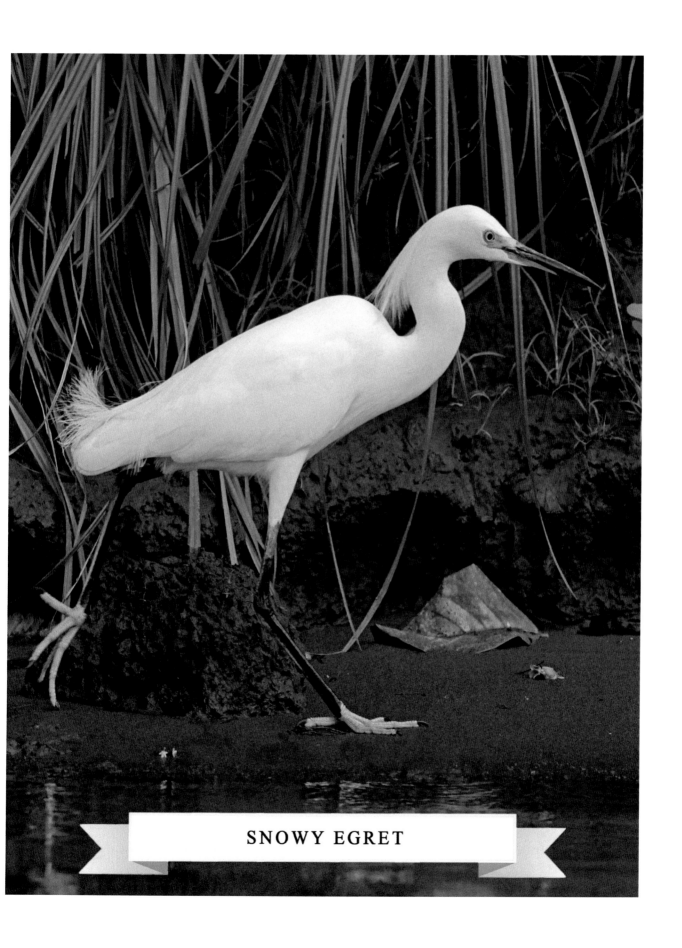

SNOWY EGRET

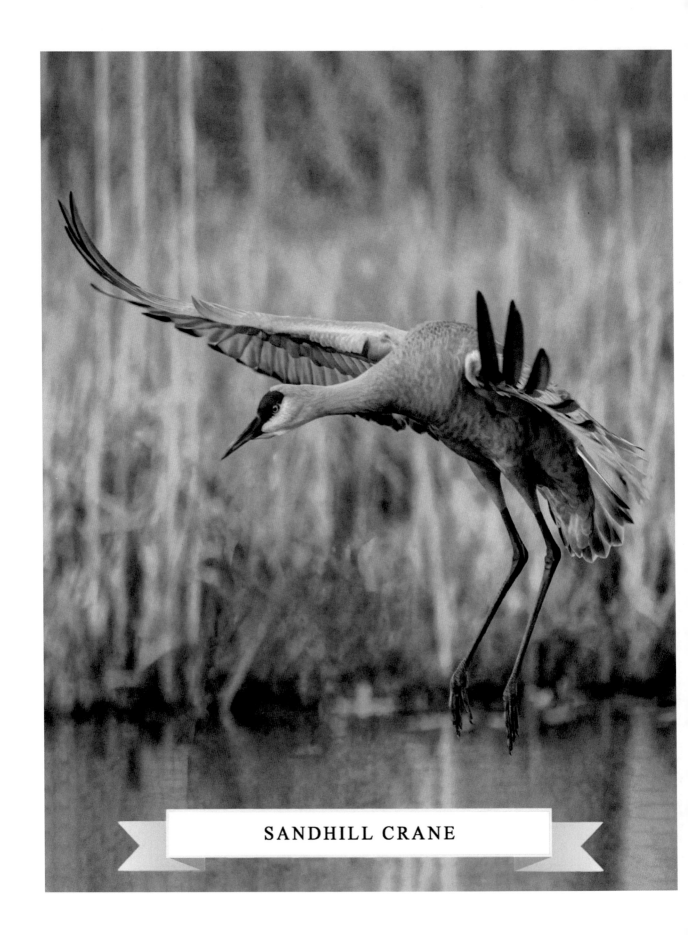

SANDHILL CRANE

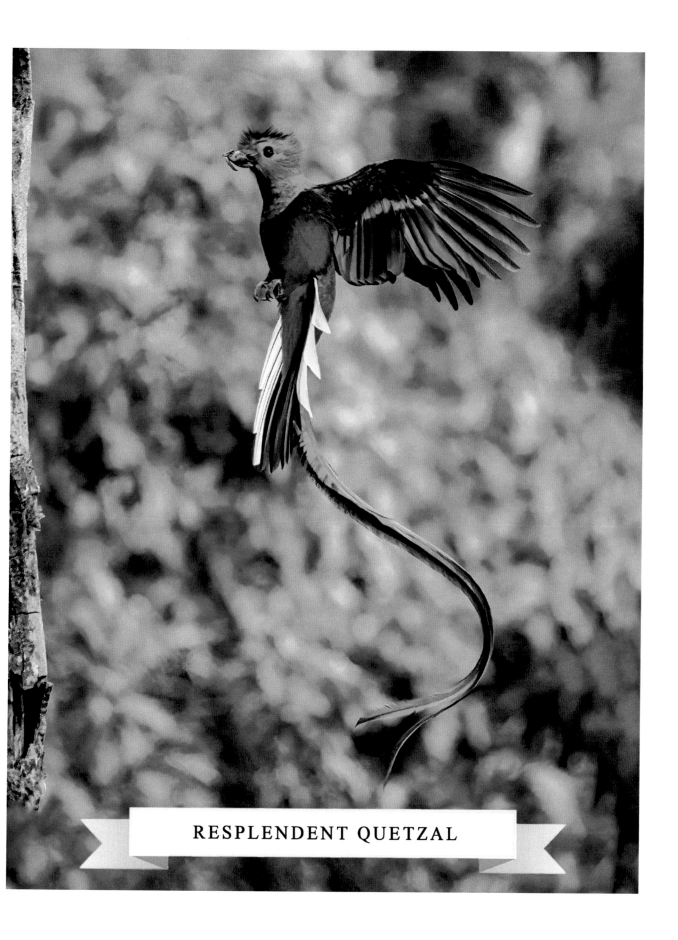

RESPLENDENT QUETZAL

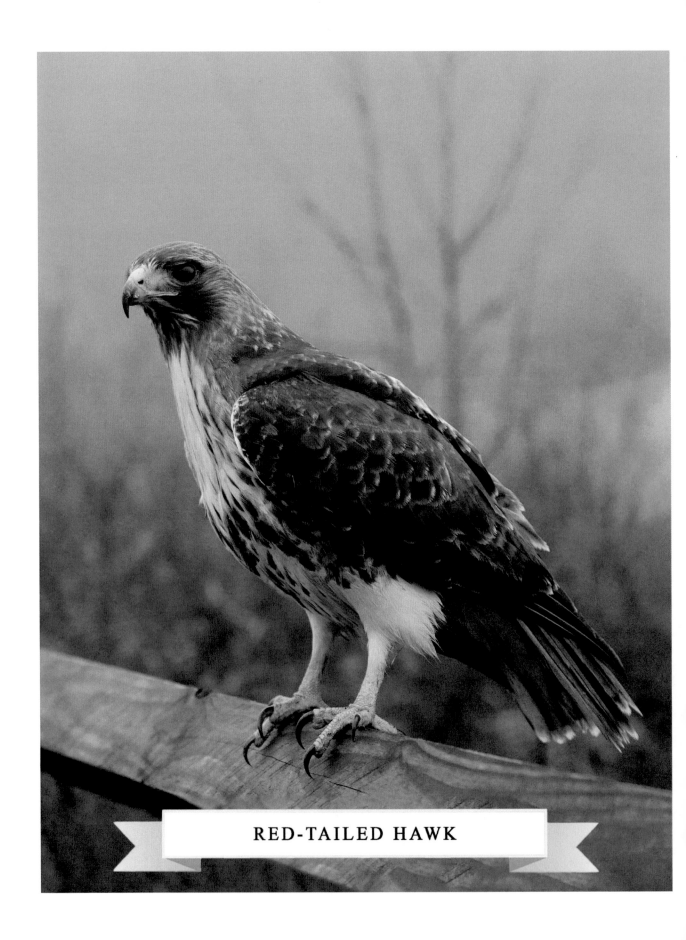

RED-TAILED HAWK

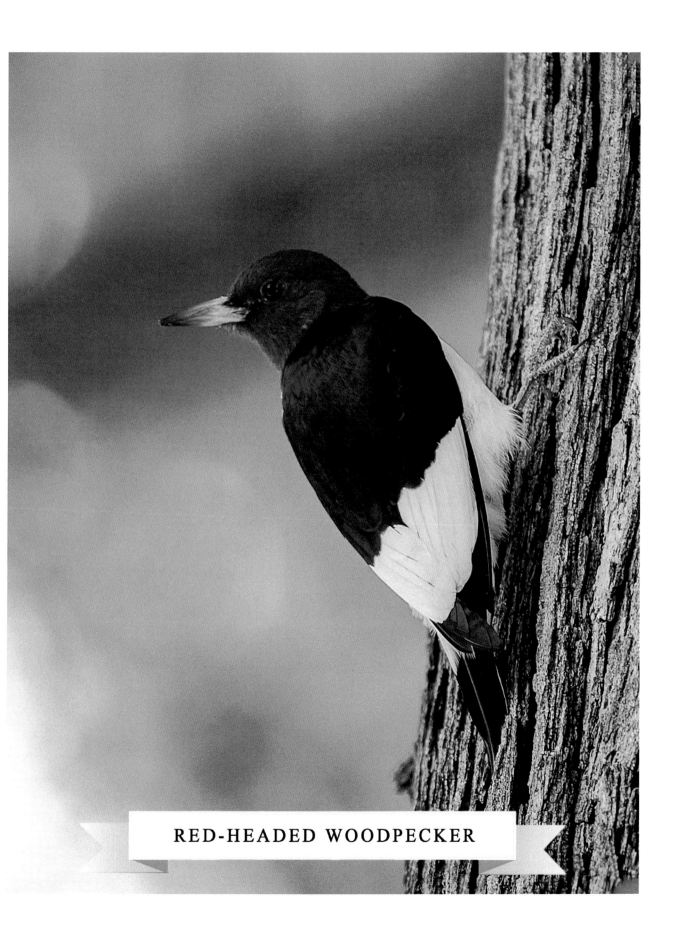

RED-HEADED WOODPECKER

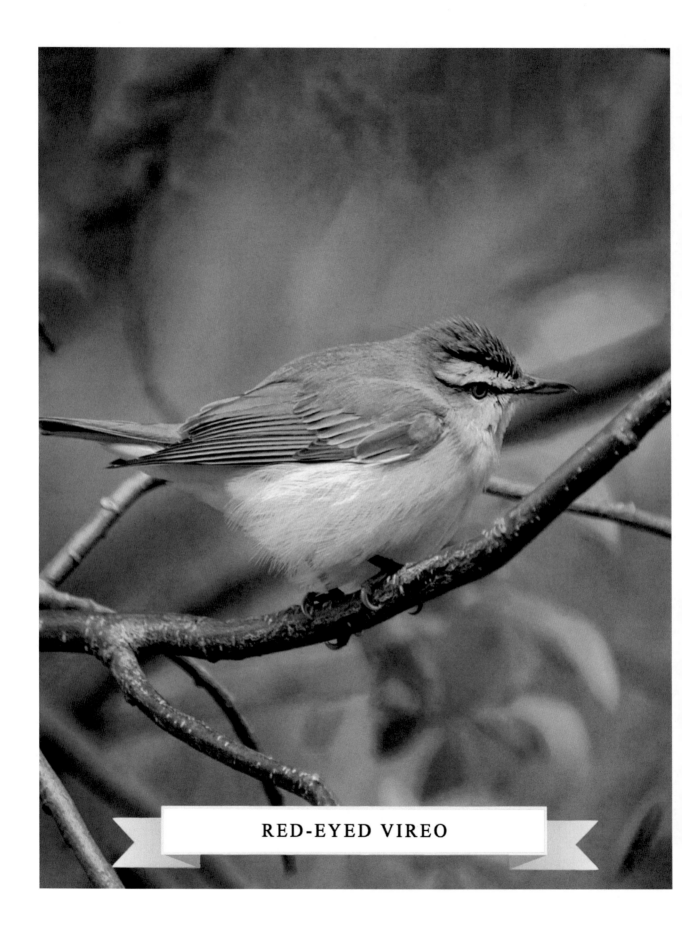

RED-EYED VIREO

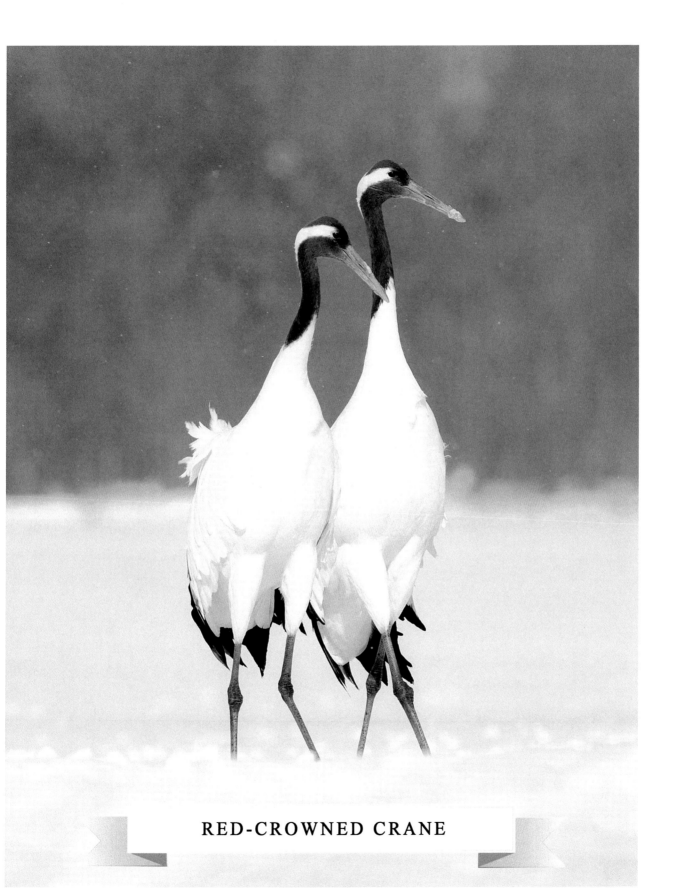

RED-CROWNED CRANE

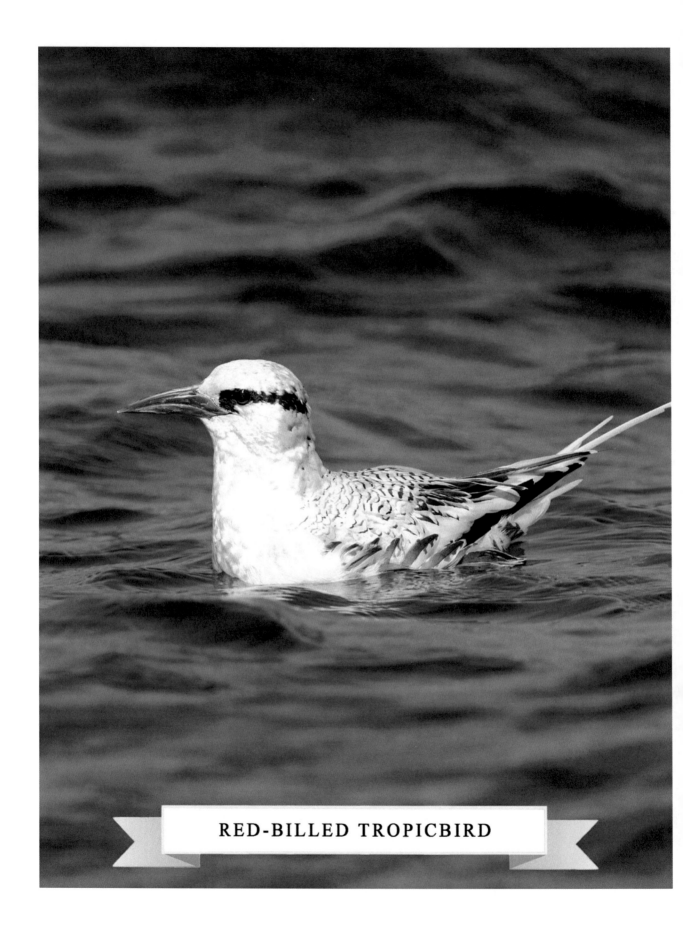

RED-BILLED TROPICBIRD

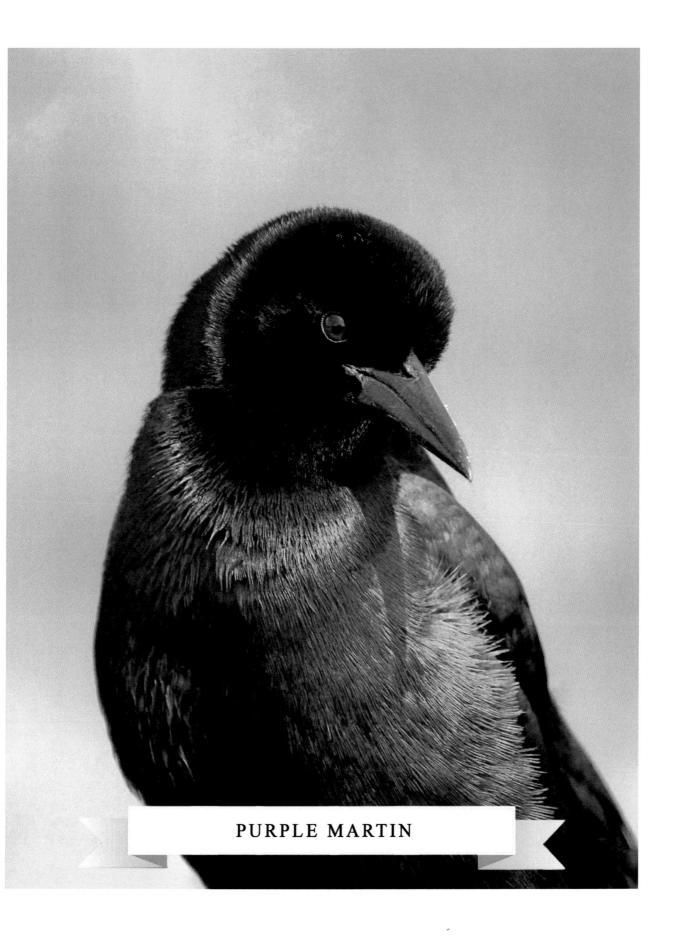

PURPLE MARTIN

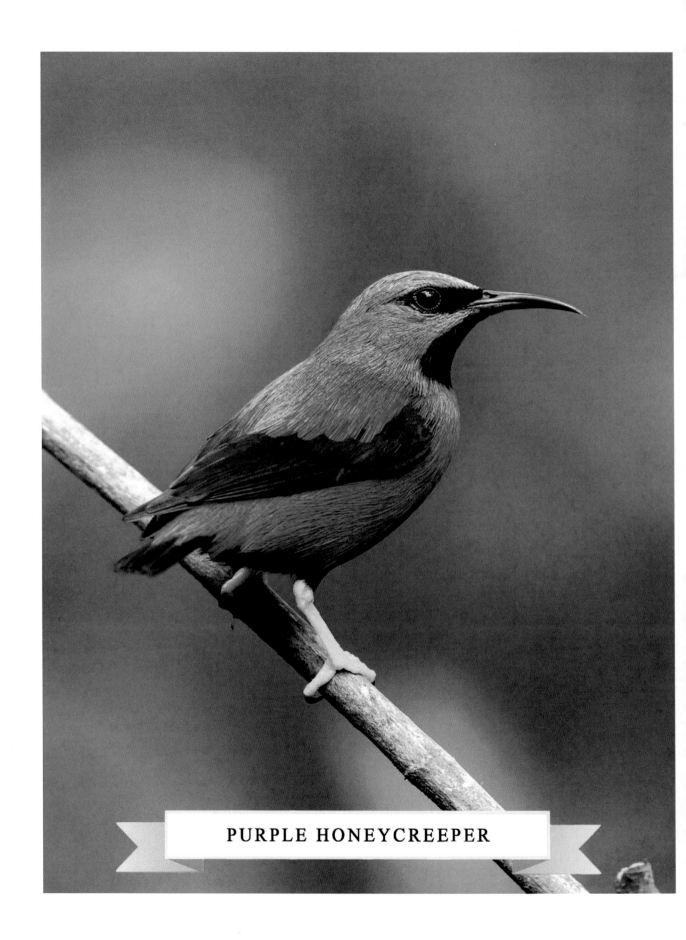

PURPLE HONEYCREEPER

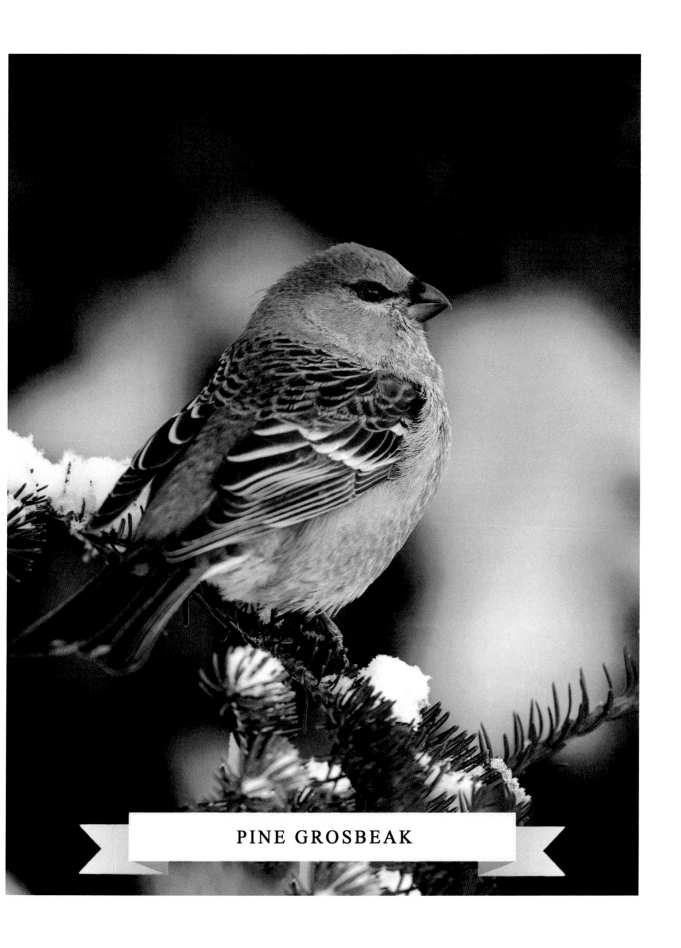

PINE GROSBEAK

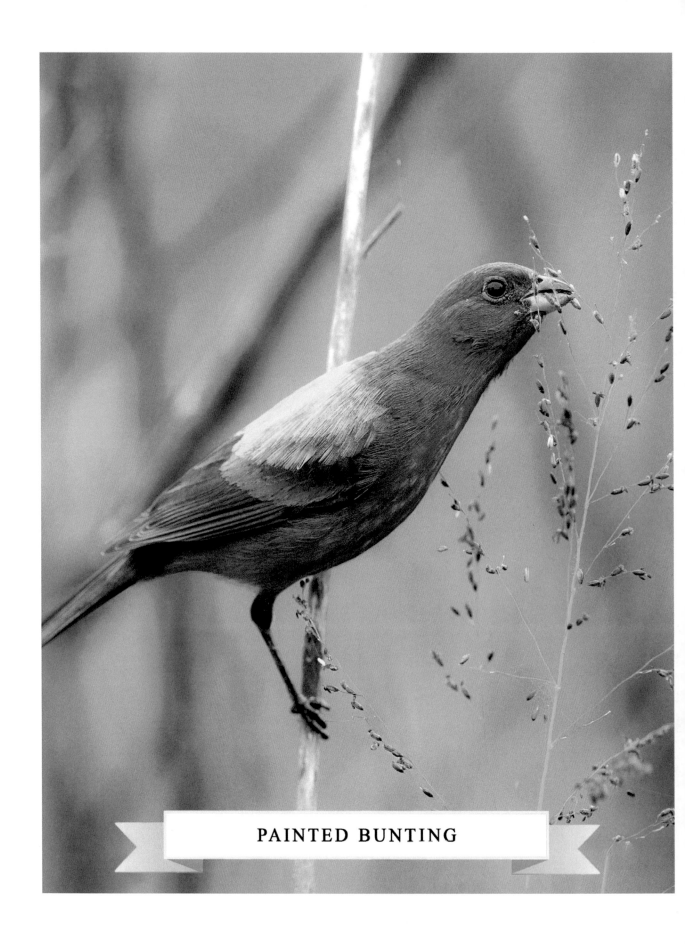

PAINTED BUNTING

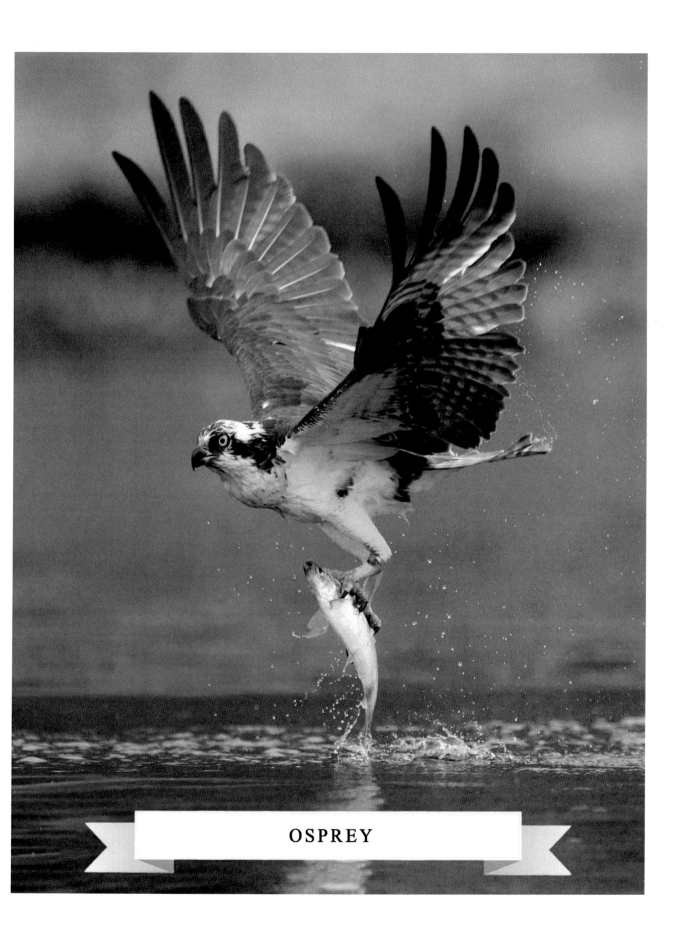

OSPREY

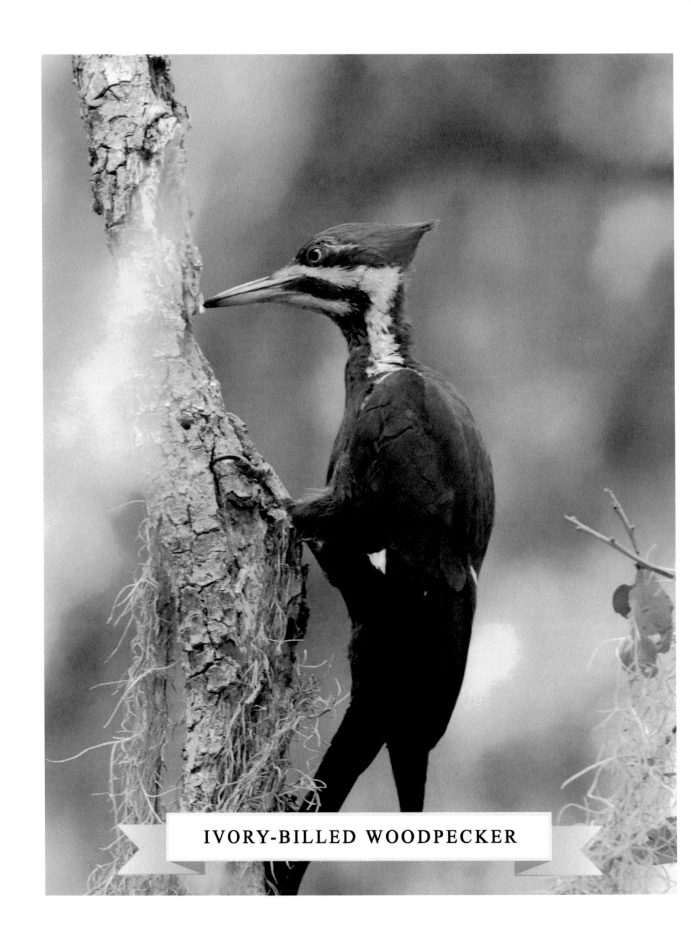

IVORY-BILLED WOODPECKER

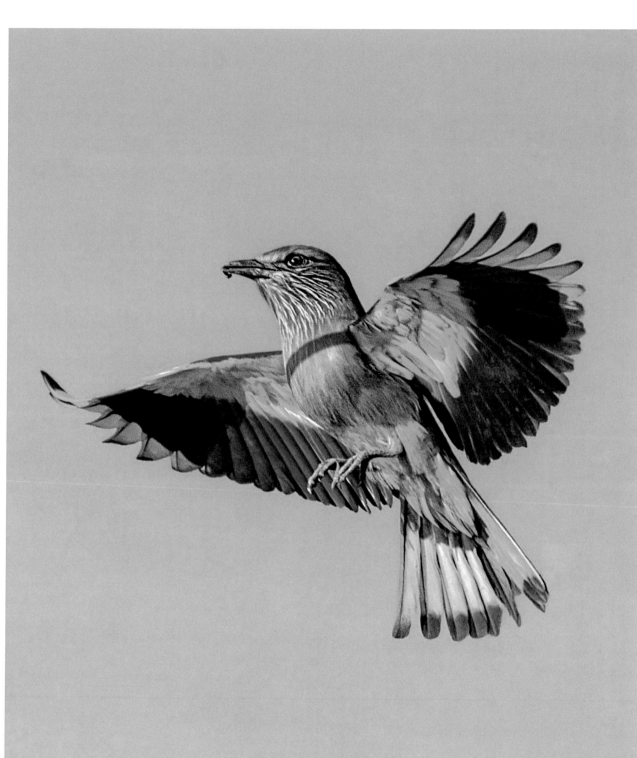

INDIAN ROLLER

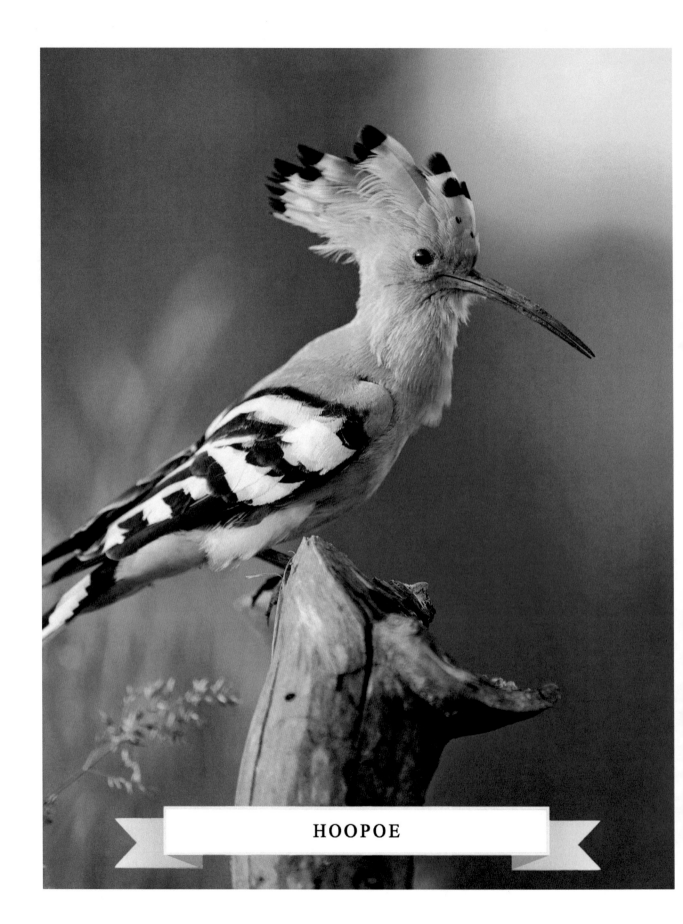

HOOPOE

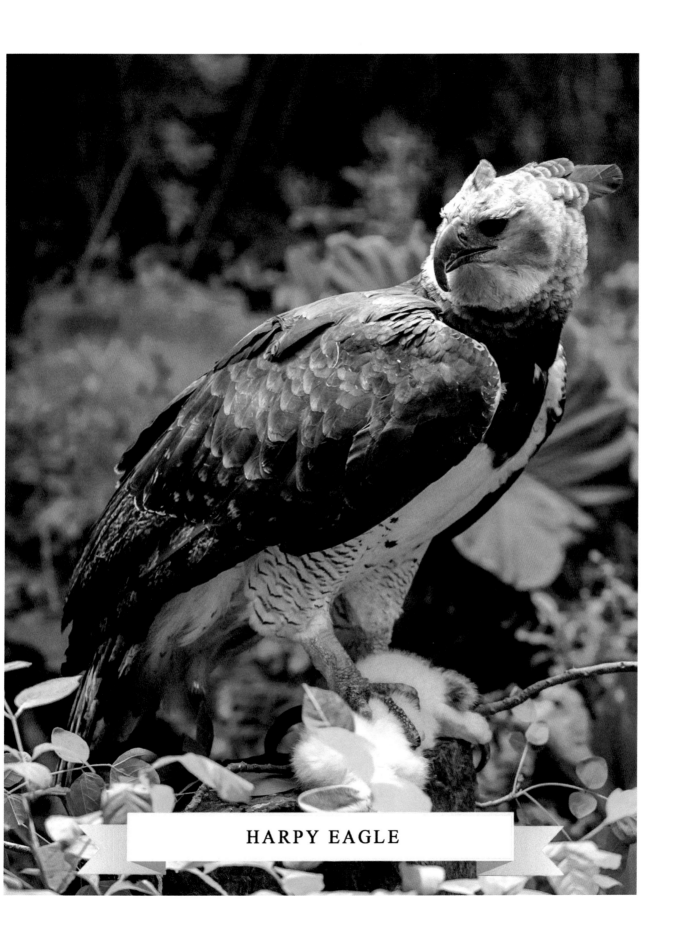

HARPY EAGLE

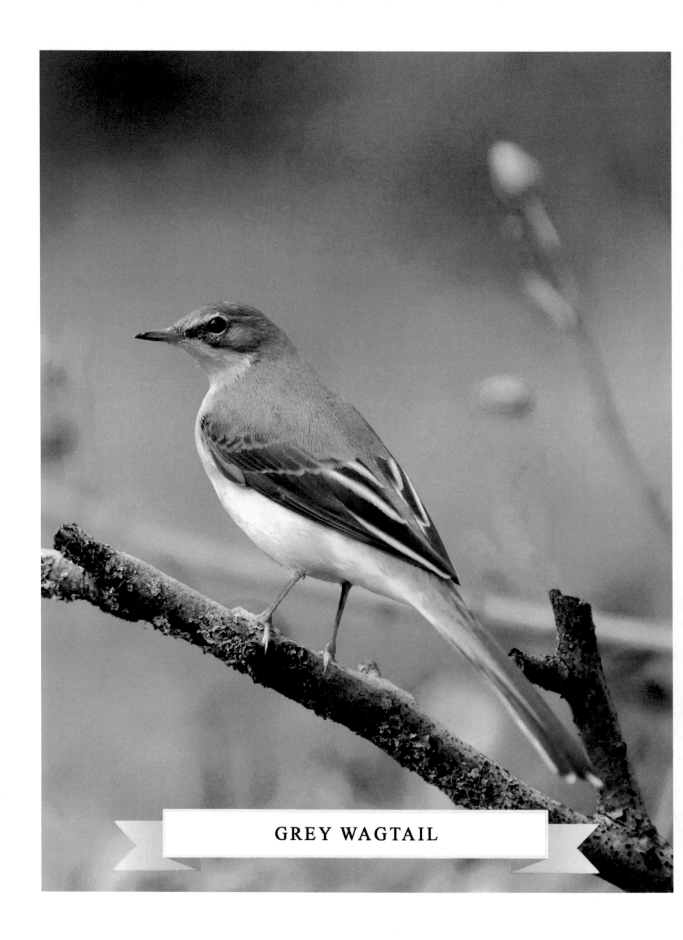

GREY WAGTAIL

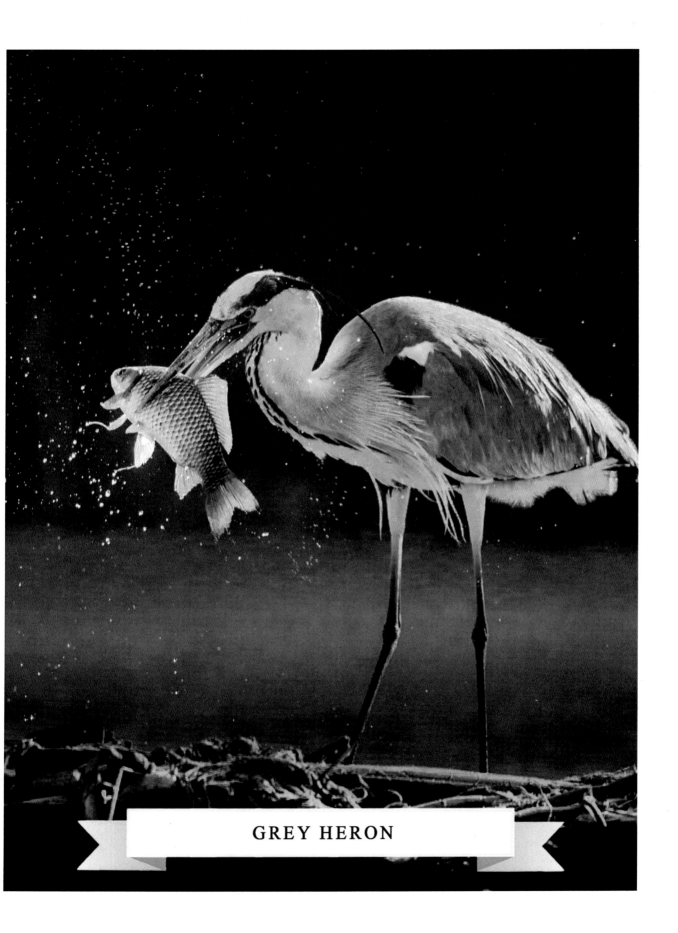

GREY HERON

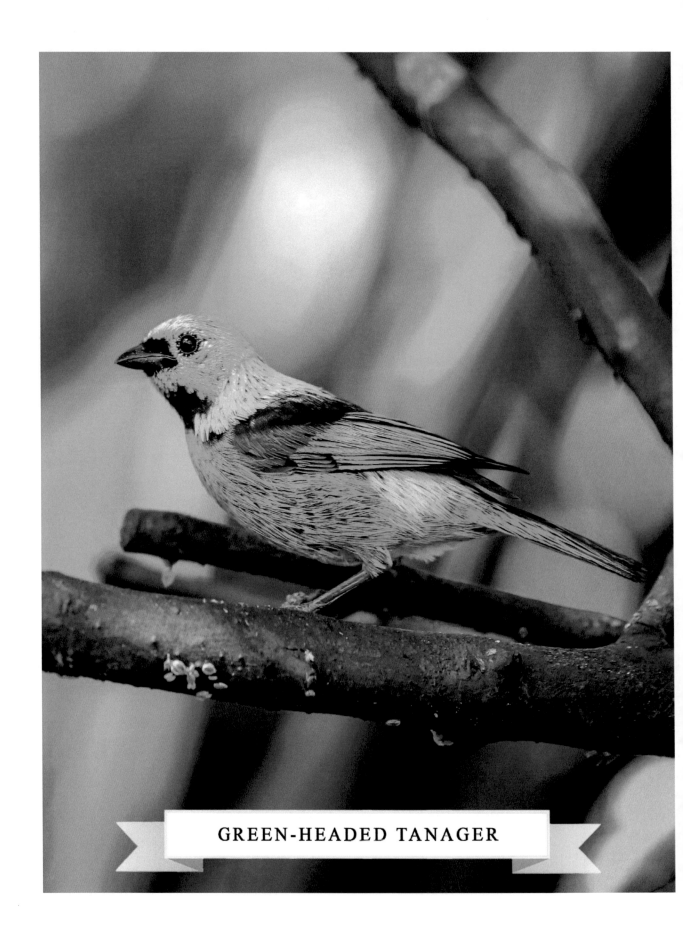

GREEN-HEADED TANAGER

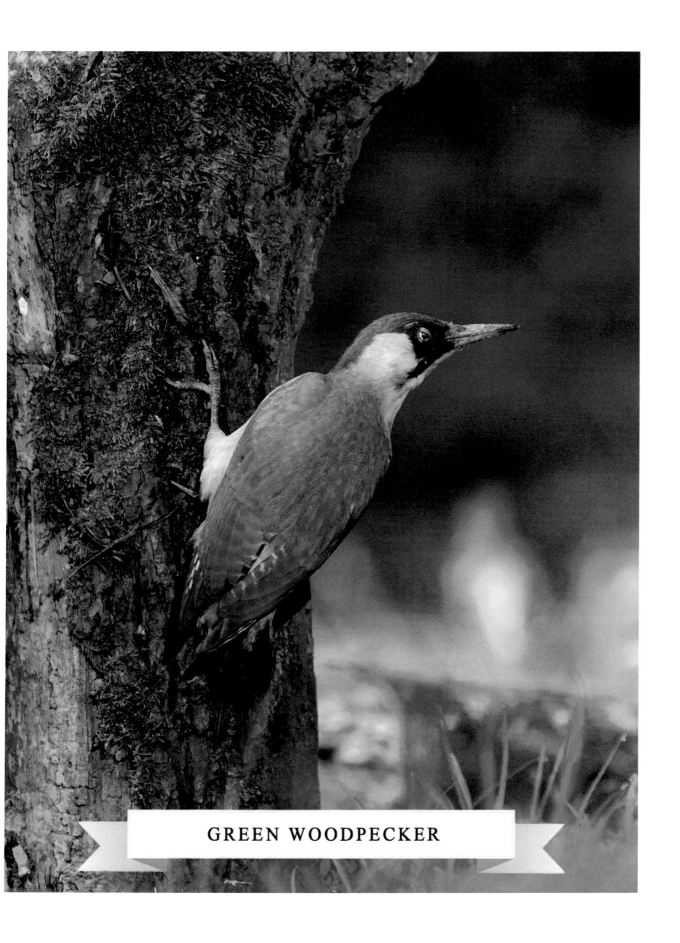

GREEN WOODPECKER

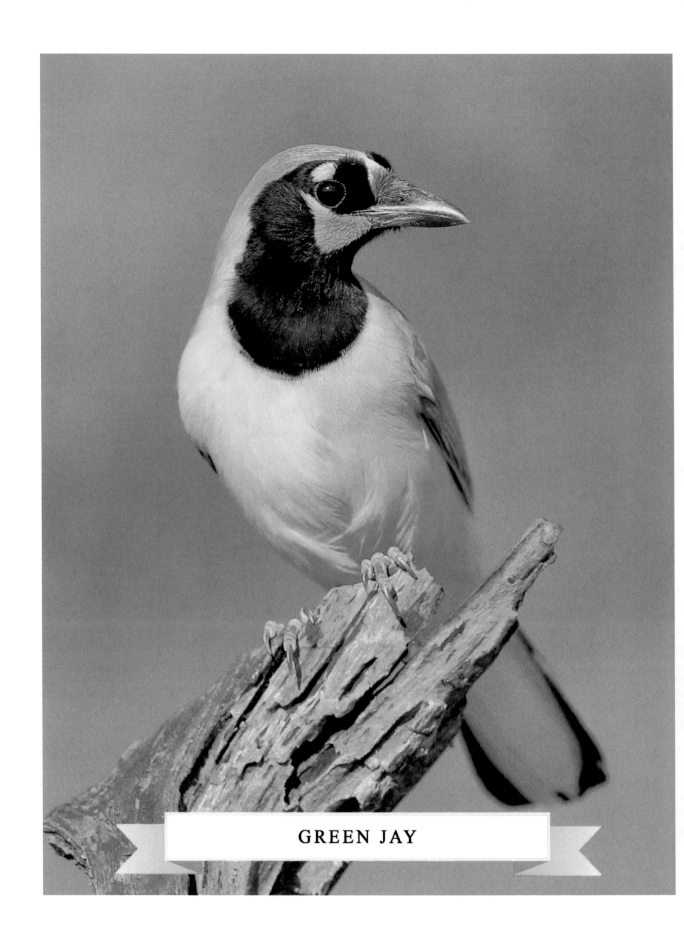

GREEN JAY

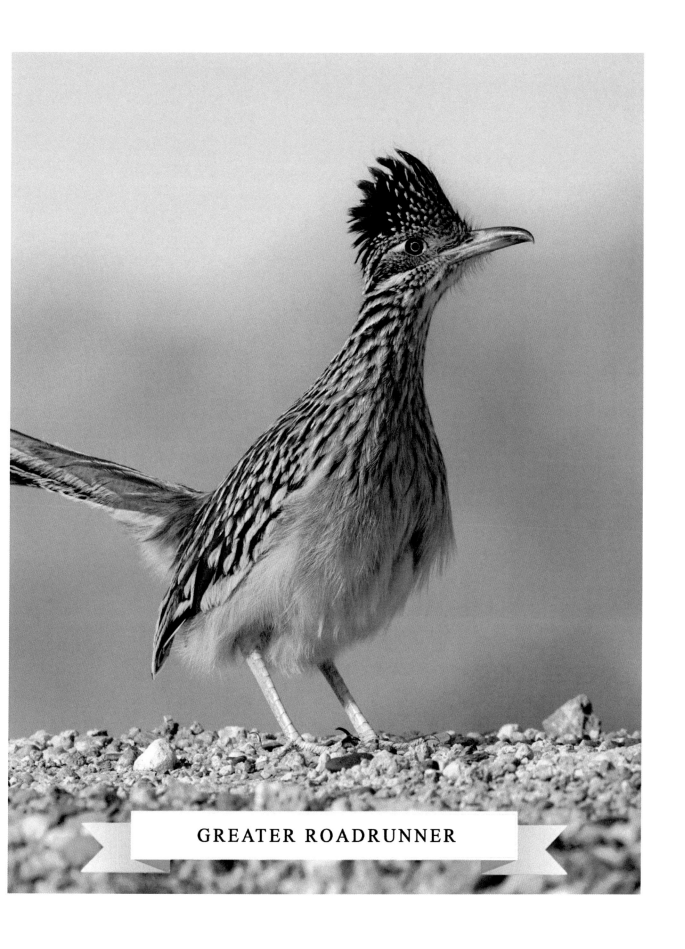

GREATER ROADRUNNER

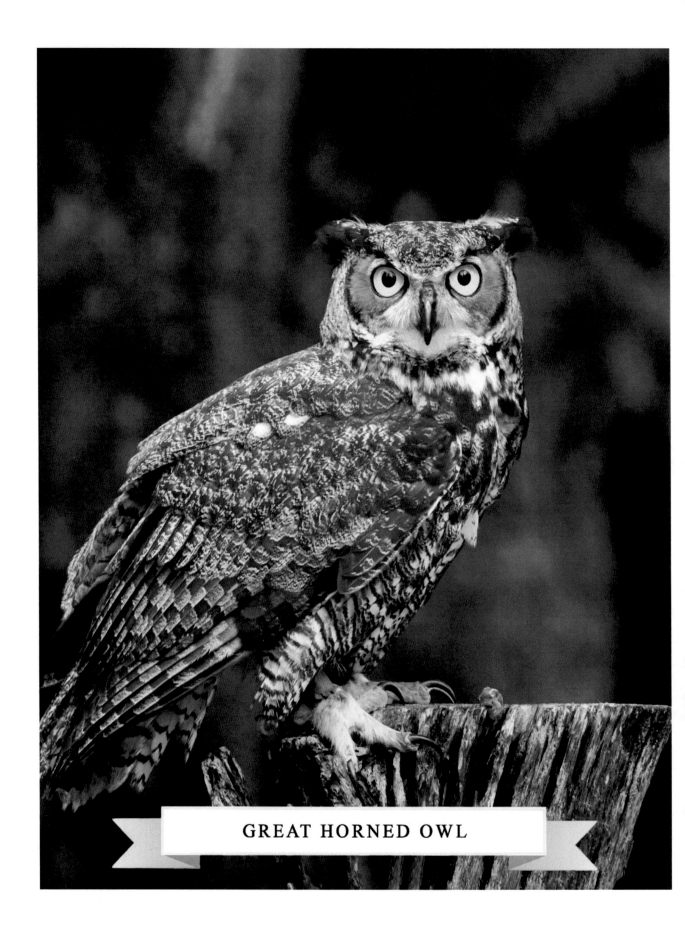

GREAT HORNED OWL

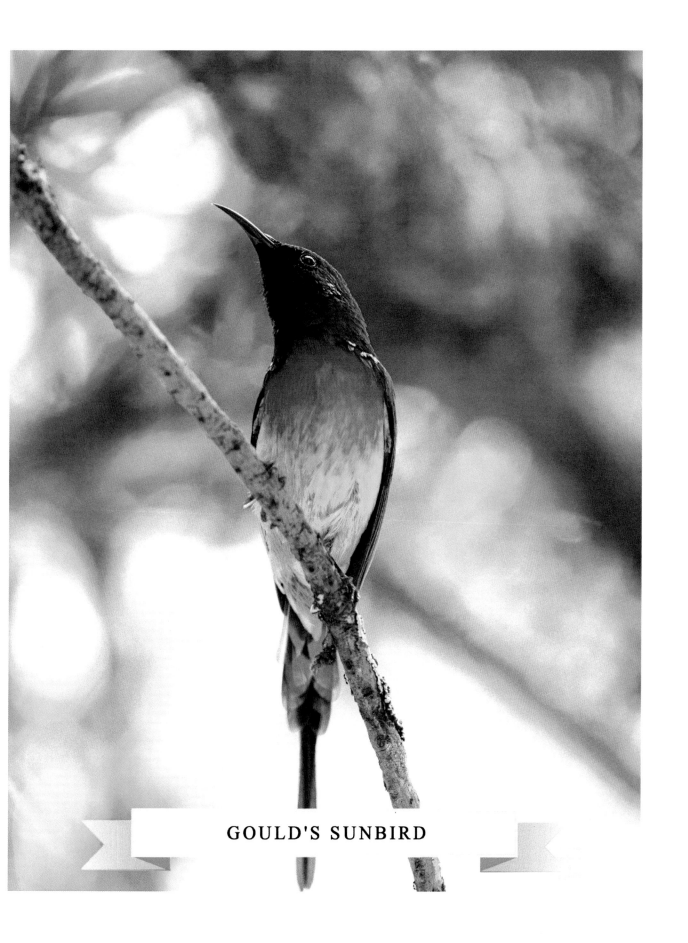

GOULD'S SUNBIRD

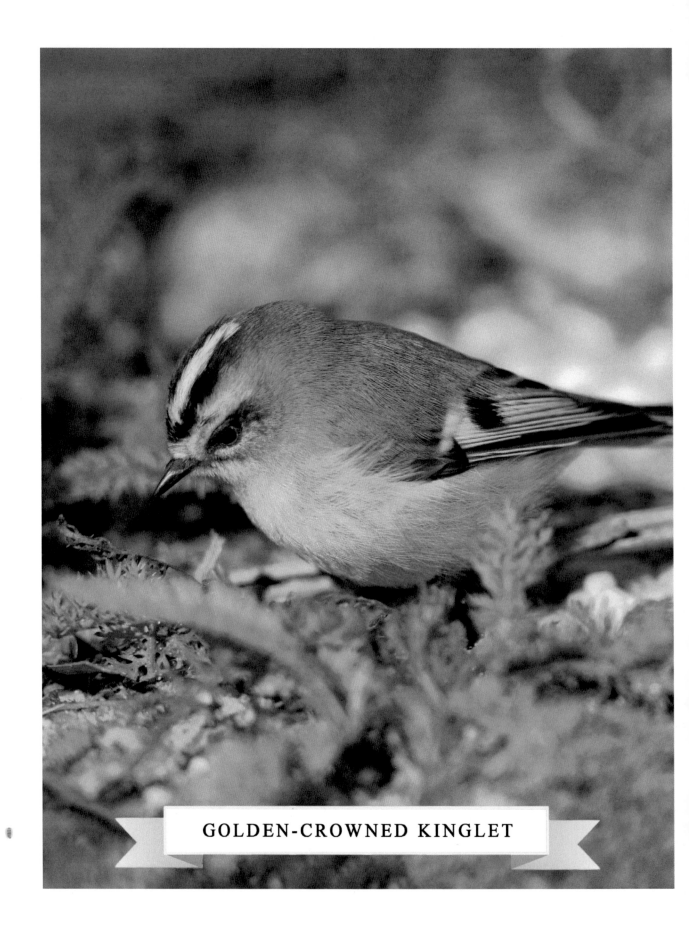

GOLDEN-CROWNED KINGLET

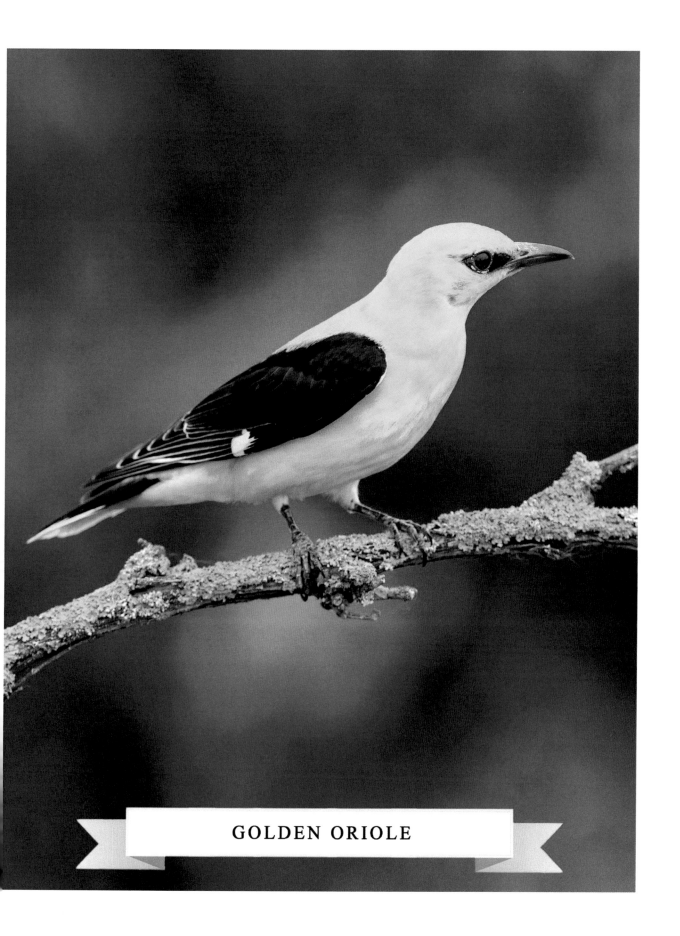

GOLDEN ORIOLE

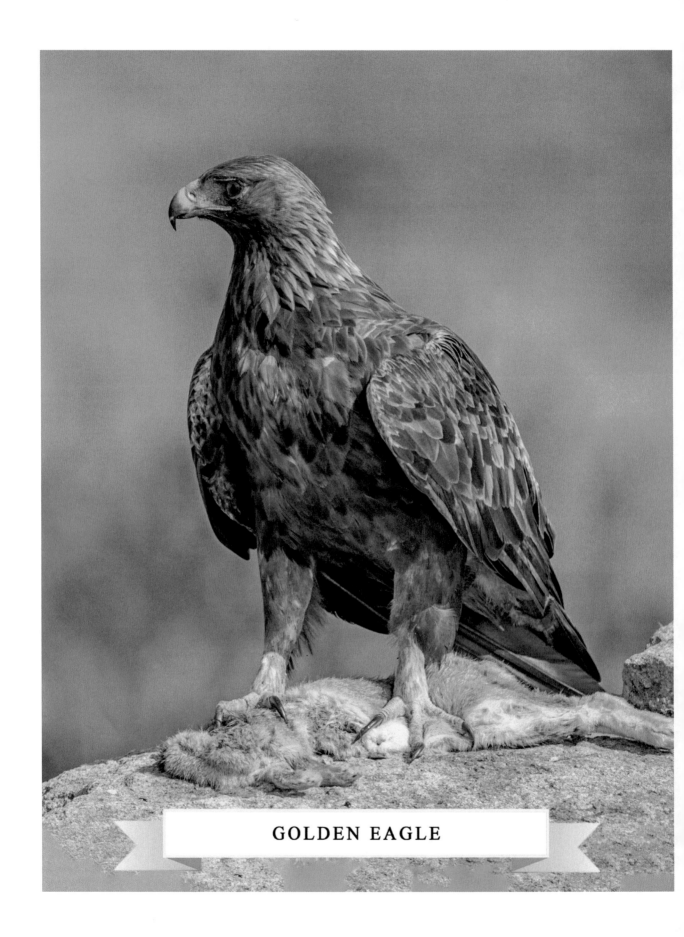

GOLDEN EAGLE

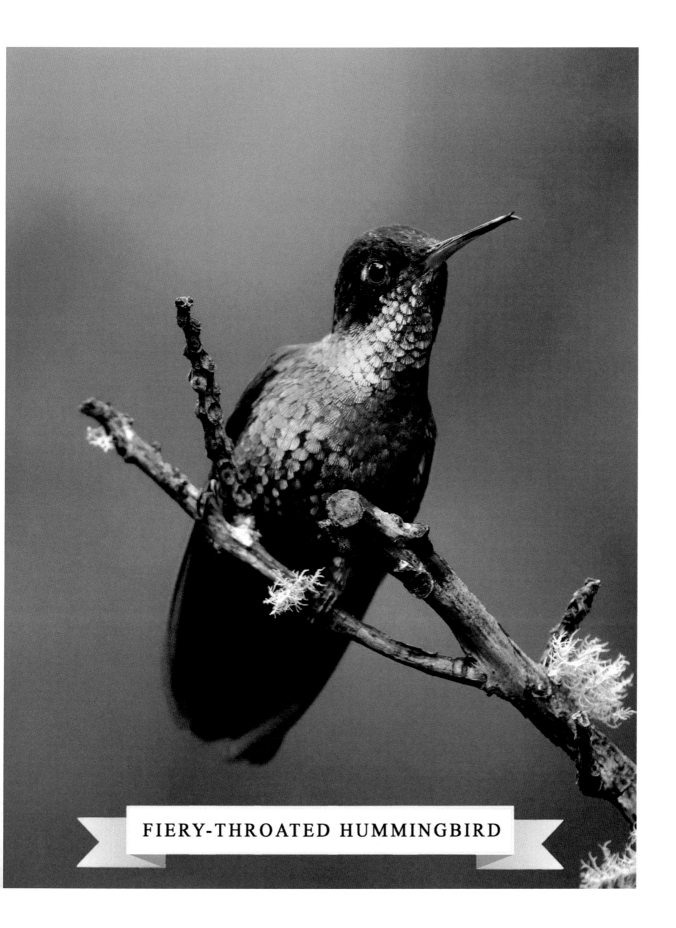

FIERY-THROATED HUMMINGBIRD

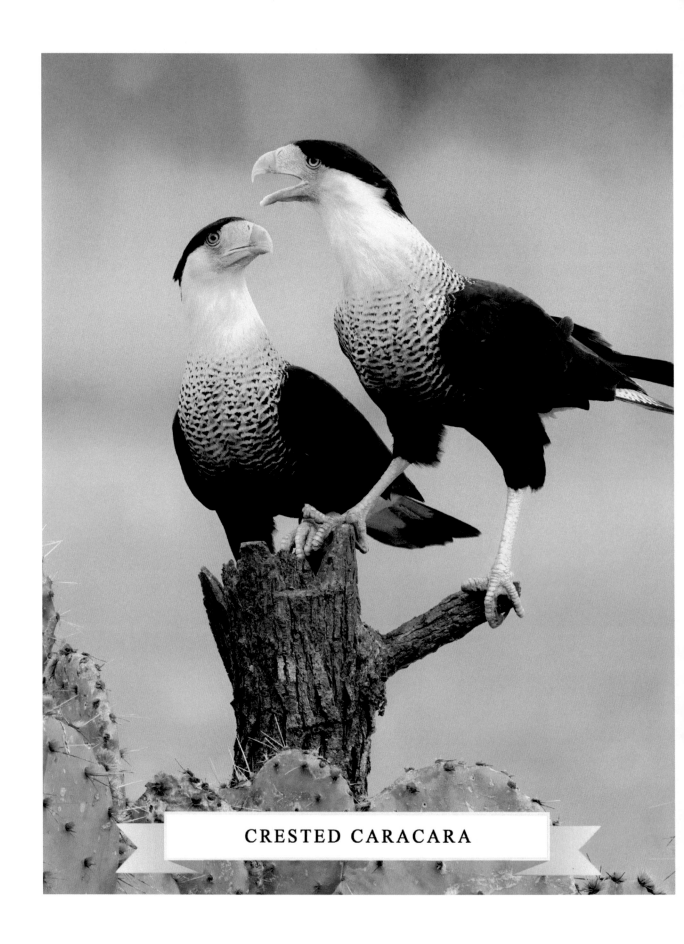

CRESTED CARACARA

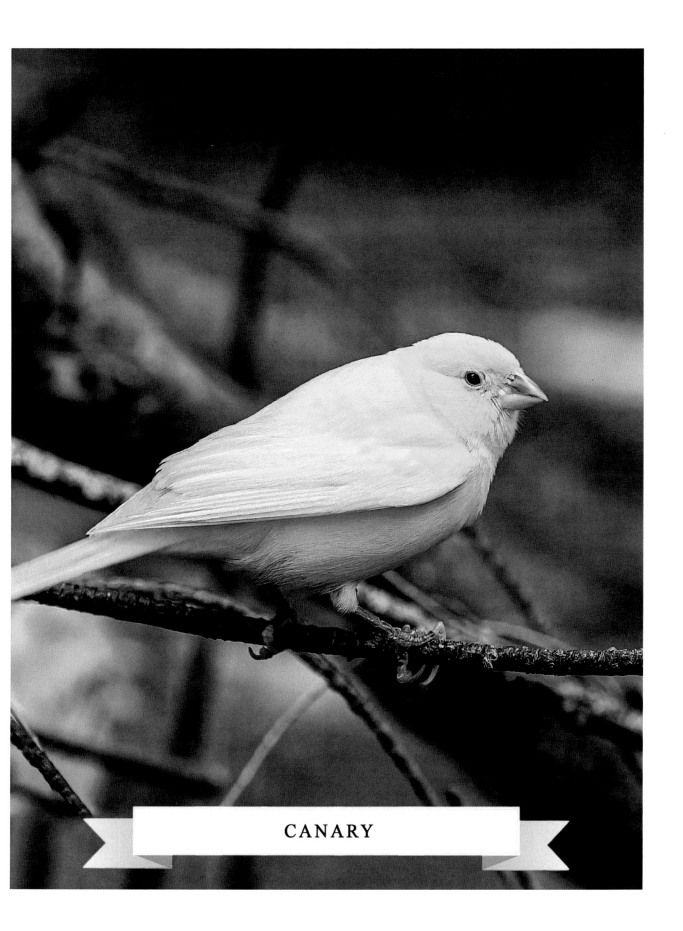

CANARY

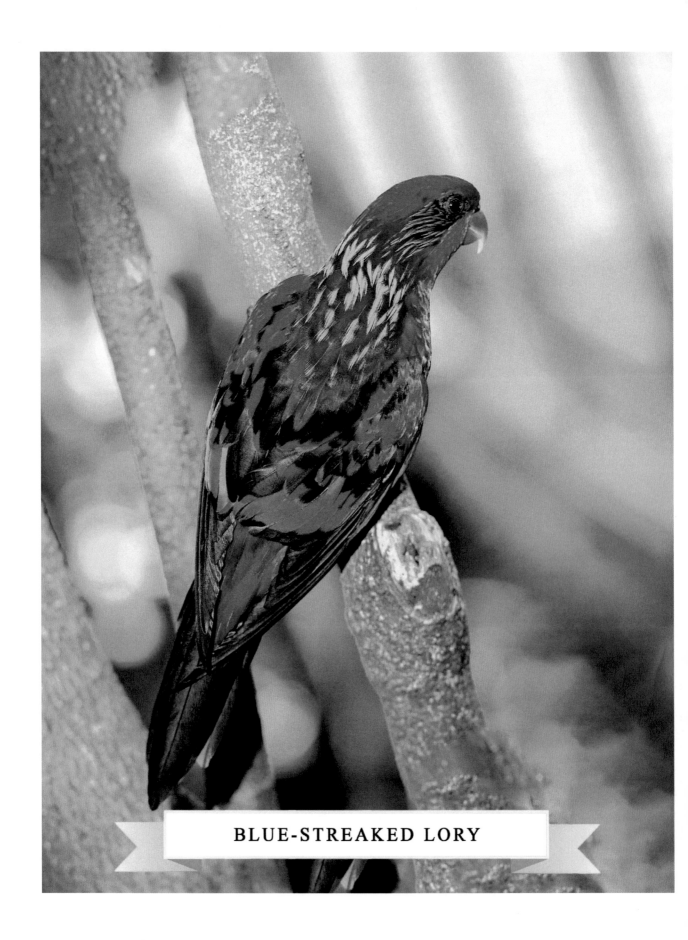

BLUE-STREAKED LORY

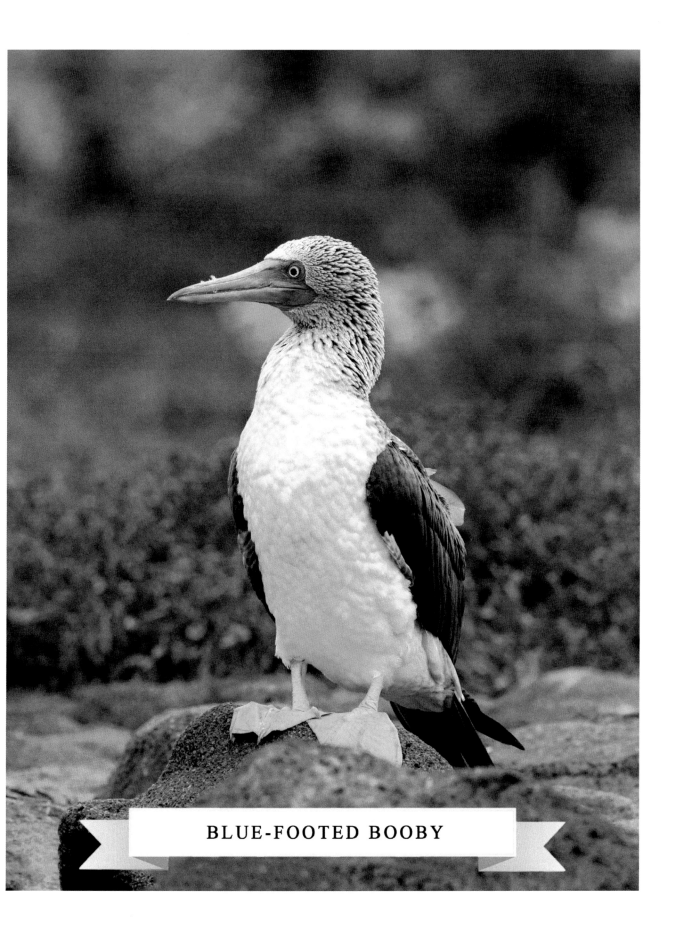

BLUE-FOOTED BOOBY

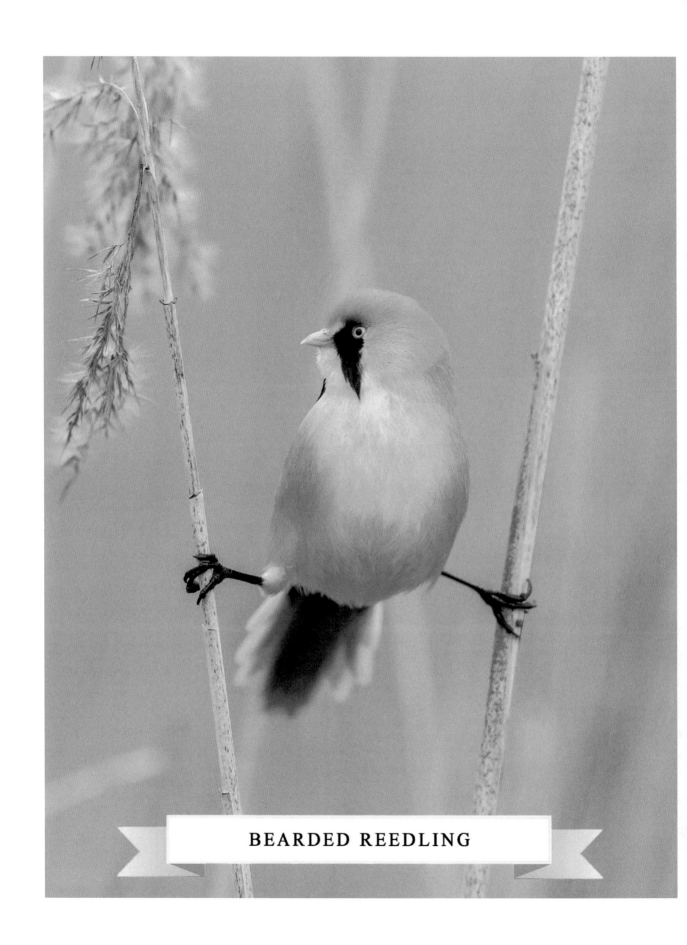

BEARDED REEDLING

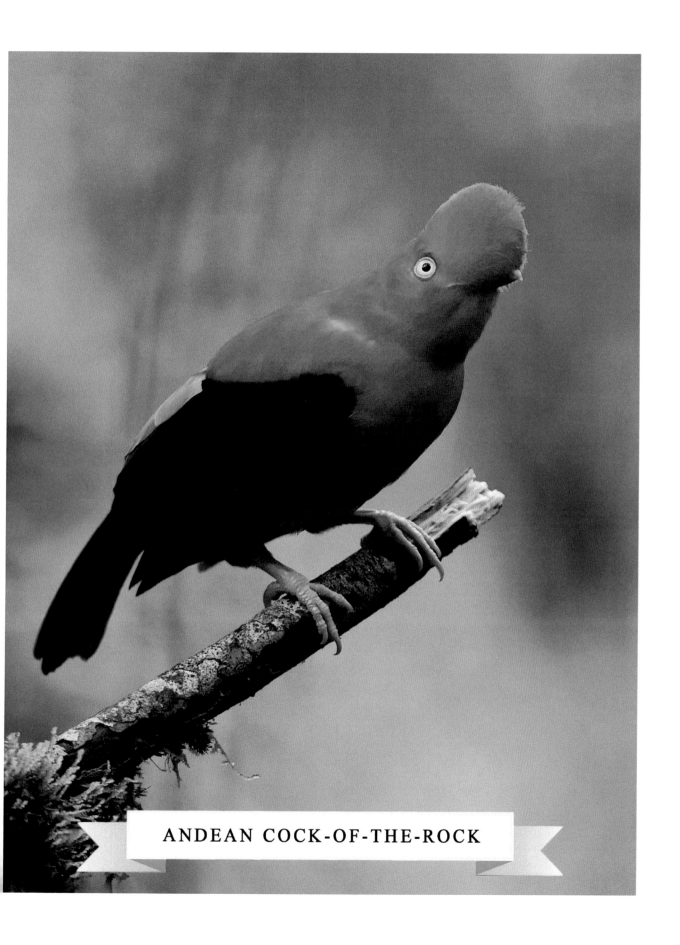

ANDEAN COCK-OF-THE-ROCK

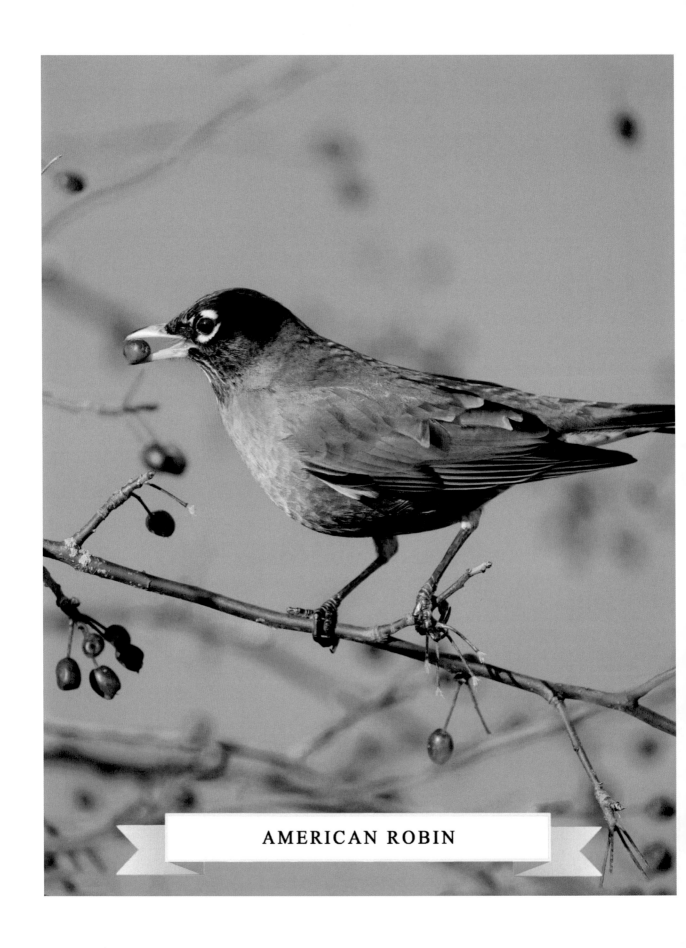

AMERICAN ROBIN

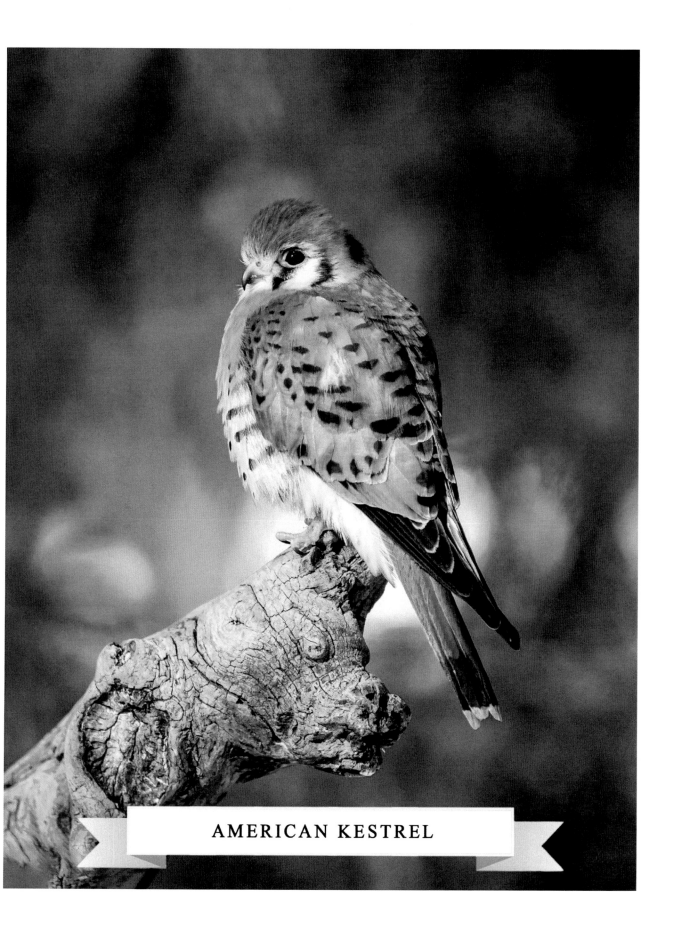

AMERICAN KESTREL

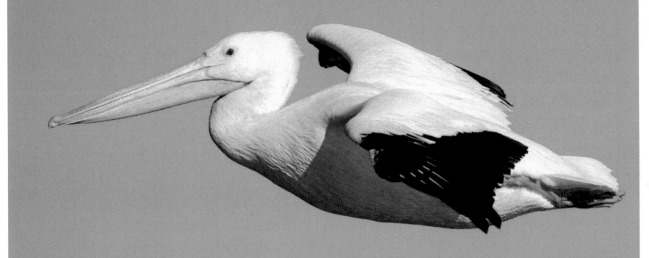

WHITE PELICAN

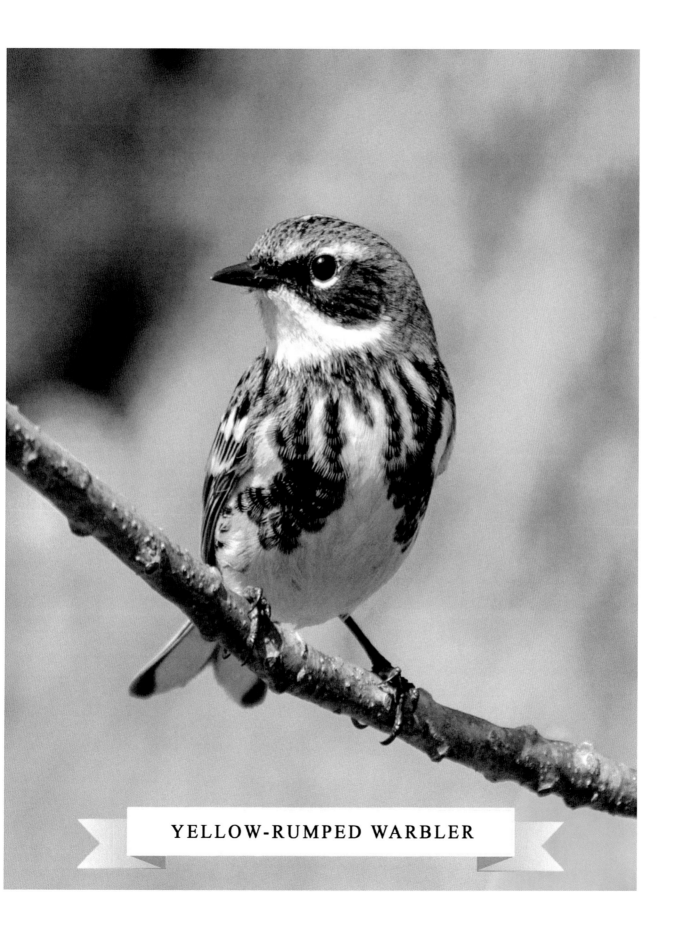

YELLOW-RUMPED WARBLER

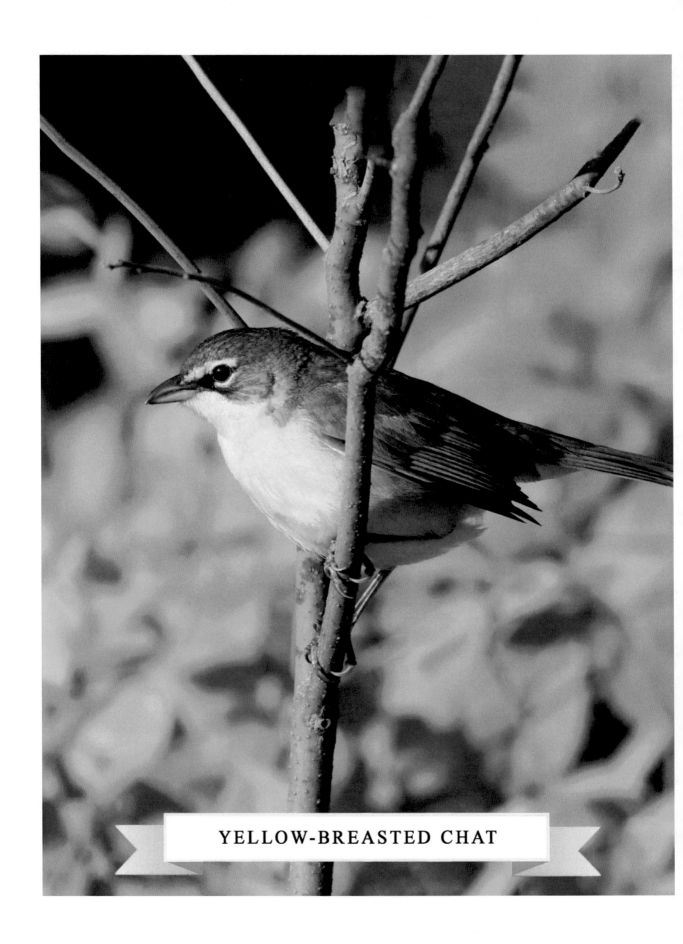

YELLOW-BREASTED CHAT

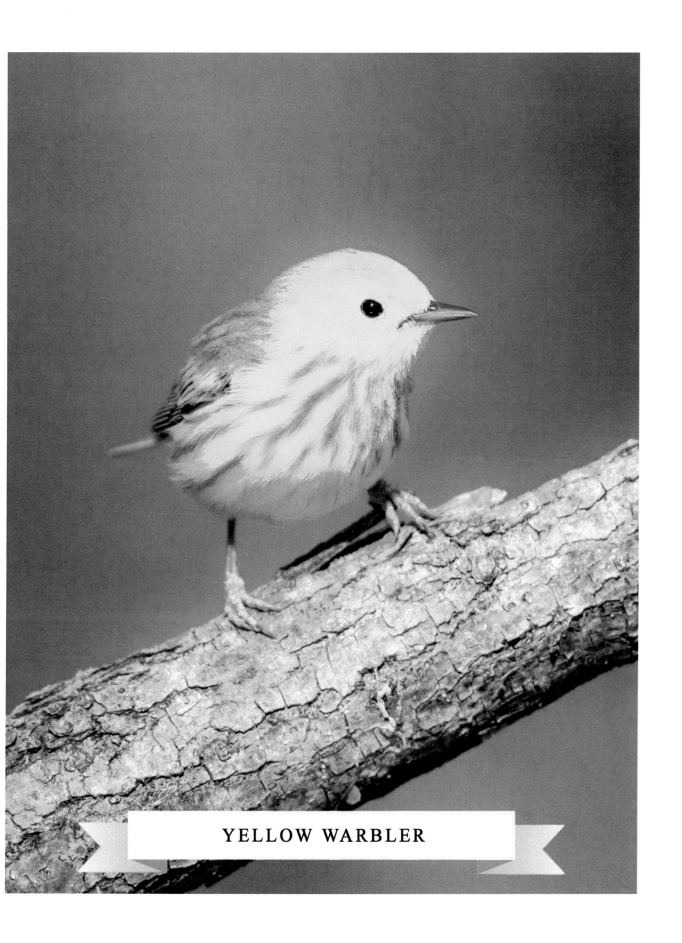

YELLOW WARBLER

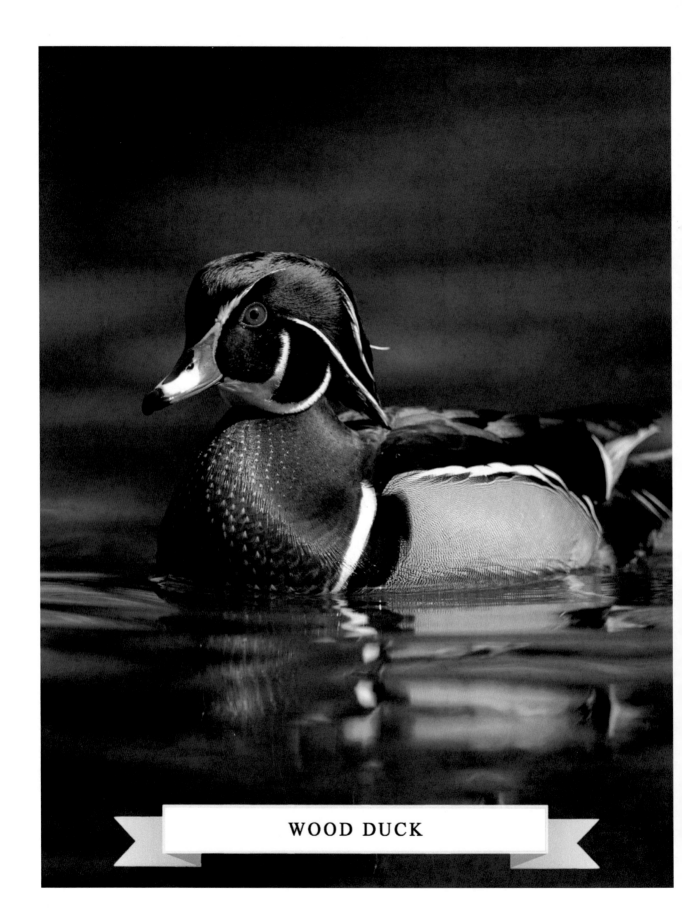

WOOD DUCK

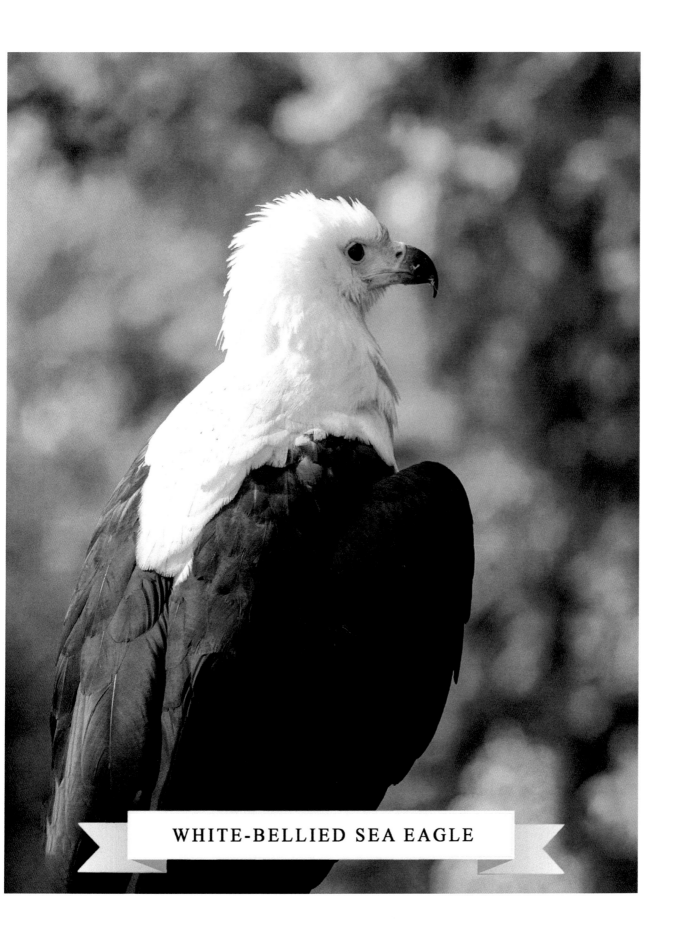

WHITE-BELLIED SEA EAGLE

Thank you

Thanks for your interest in our books.

Please consider purchasing our other books
available now at Amazon.com.

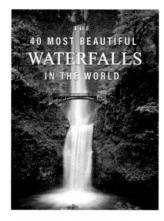
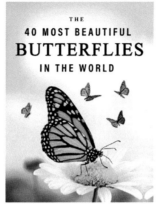
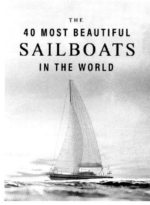
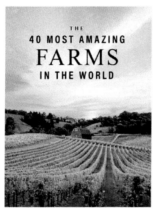

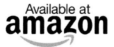

(Just search for "Blue Clover Books" on Amazon.)

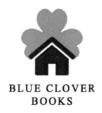

Made in the USA
Las Vegas, NV
07 May 2024

89616471R00062